OMT REVIEW

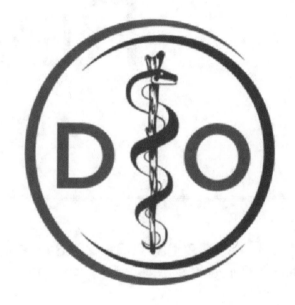

4th Edition

Editor-in-chief

Robert G. Savarese DO

OMT
REVIEW
4th EDITION

Copyright © 1998, 1999, 2003, 2009, 2018 by Robert G. Savarese, D.O.
Chapter 13 "Lymphatics" Copyright © by John D. Capobianco, D.O. F.A.A.O. printed with permission.

For any comments, questions, and suggestions,
please send e-mail to the author at omtreview@hotmail.com

Reprints of chapters may be purchased from
Robert Savarese at <u>omtreview@hotmail.com</u>

ISBN: 978-0-692-15756-5
Printed in the United States of America

<u>Notice</u>: The authors of this volume have taken care to make certain that the information contained herein is correct and compatible with the standards generally accepted at the time of the publication. As new information becomes available, changes in treatment modalities invariably follow; therefore when choosing a particular treatment, the reader should consider not only the information provided in this manual but also any recently published medical literature on the subject. The nature of this text is to be a comprehensive review, but due to the extraordinary amount of material it is beyond the scope of this text to include all aspects of osteopathic medicine. It is advised that the reader familiarizes himself with the information contained in one of the excellent osteopathic texts that form the cornerstone of osteopathic medical education. Lastly, the authors and distributors disclaim any liability, loss, injury, or damage incurred as a consequence, directly or indirectly, of the use and application from any of the contents of this volume.

Editor-in-chief

Robert Savarese DO
Jacksonville Orthopaedic Institute
Baptist Medical Center
Jacksonville, Florida

Illustration Editor/Question Bank Developer/Editor

Adeleke Adesina DO
Emergency Medicine
Methodist Hospital
Houston, Texas
Founder, Ftplectures.com

Question Editor/Q Bank Editor

Grant Reed, DO
Family Medicine
St. Margaret's Health Center
Peru, Illinois

Assistant Editors

John D. Capobianco, DO, FAAO
Clinical Associate Professor
Department of Osteopathic Medicine
New York Institute of Technology College of Osteopathic Medicine
Old Westbury, New York

Jennifer Savarese, MD
Private Practice
Jacksonville Pediatrics
Jacksonville, Florida

Chapter Contributors

Glenn Fuoco, DO (Special Tests - Chapter 18)
Daniel Berson, DO (Muscle Energy - Chapter 15)
John Capobianco.DO (Lymphatics - Chapter 13)

Dedication

To my loving wife, Jennifer, and my daughters.
Without your loving support this 4th edition of our book would not have
been possible.

– Robert Savarese, DO

To the the Almighty God, who has granted me life and the opportunity to
contribute to the 4th edition of this book. I also want to thank the love of
my life Olufunmilayo and my sons, Olamide and Oluwadamola Adesina
for their ever loving support of me.

– Adeleke Adesina, DO

Preface

It's hard to believe that over twenty years ago, while studying for my COMLEX® level 1 that I discovered the need for a comprehensive OMT Review book. Back then, thousands of students including myself, were left sifting through two years of OMT notes, or reading various texts, in order to study for the OMT section of the boards. . With each of the three editions, the book has gained success and I would like to personally thank the osteopathic community for supporting OMT Review.

Several years have elapsed since the last edition. Therefore, I felt that it was important to revise all of the content to reflect the current understanding and knowledge of osteopathic medicine as written in the Foundations for Osteopathic Medicine and the many other texts that form the cornerstone of osteopathic medical education.

Technology has advanced tremendously since the third edition of OMT Review. Today's medical students' are more connected and require information at their fingertips. We wanted to provide our osteopathic medical students online access. This is why we have removed the COMLEX-style questions located at the end of previous editions and migrated them to an online version that is similar to the COMLEX® question bank interface. This service is FREE for students that purchased an OMT Review 4TH Edition book. Use the scratch-off code on the inside cover, to create an account and receive over 300 revised OMM questions for free. The new OMT Review question bank covers not only provides OMM questions, but for a monthly subscription, students can practice all subjects commonly tested on the COMLEX® exam. Students will be able to log on and take thousands of practice test questions online, see their results compared to their peers. The new OMT Review question bank was developed to help students

improve their knowledge, gauge their progress and pass
the COMLEX® exam.

You can register online to access the question bank on

OMTReview.net

The website also provides OMT review COMLEX-
style videos covering all high yield concepts tested on the
OMT portion on the COMLEX® exam and OMT review
flashcards to help the student for last minute review
during board preparation.

OMT Review is not intended to substitute for any of
the excellent osteopathic reference texts. It is intended
to be used as quick reference as well as a board review.
A combination of basic osteopathic principles along with
important clinical points makes this book useful for
osteopathic medical students as well as anyone
interested in osteopathic medicine. It is hoped that the
concise style, tables, and illustrations help summarize
and enhance the readers' recollection of principle points.

It is my sincere wish that this book will serve as a
resource through which its readers can rapidly grasp the
fundamental principles of osteopathic medicine.

Robert G. Savarese DO

*The COMLEX-USA examinations are developed, administered and owned by the National Board
of Osteopathic Medical Examiners Inc. (NBOME). COMLEX® and COMLEX-USA® are registered
trademarks of NBOME.*

Table of Contents

CHAPTER 14 COUNTERSTRAIN AND FACILITATED POSITIONAL RELEASE

CHAPTER 15 MUSCLE ENERGY

CHAPTER 16 HIGH VELOCITY LOW AMPLITUDE (HVLA)

CHAPTER 17 ARTICULATORY TECHNIQUES

CHAPTER 18 SPECIAL TESTS

APPENDIX A COMMON TECHNIQUES FOR VISCERAL AND SYSTEMIC DYSFUNCTION

APPENDIX B NEUROLOGIC EXAM

The Basics 1

I. Somatic dysfunction

A. Definition – *"Somatic dysfunction is an impairment or altered function of related components of the somatic (body framework) system: skeletal, arthroidial, and myofascial structures and related vascular, lymphatic and neural elements."* [1 p.1106]

In simpler terms: Somatic dysfunction is a restriction that can occur in bones joints, muscle, and fascia. Blood supply, lymph flow and nervous function may be altered in somatic dysfunction.

B. Diagnostic criteria

A somatic dysfunction can present as:

1. <u>Tissue texture changes</u> – may present in many ways. The surrounding tissue may be edematous, tender, fibrosed, atrophied, rigid, or hypertonic.

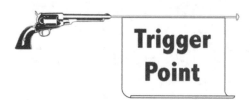

Trigger Point

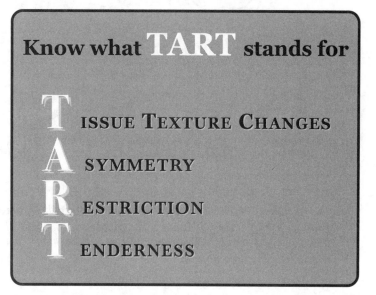

Know what **TART** stands for

Tissue Texture Changes

Asymmetry

Restriction

Tenderness

2. <u>Asymmetry</u> – bones, muscles, or joints may feel asymmetric to the corresponding structures.

3. <u>Restriction</u> (see Figure 1.1a and 1.1b) – a joint with a somatic dysfunction will have restricted motion. Under normal physiologic conditions a joint has two barriers:

   a. **Physiologic barrier** – a point at which a patient can actively move any given joint. For example, a person may actively rotate his head 80° to either side.

   b. **Anatomic barrier** – a point at which a physician can passively move any given joint. For example, a physician may passively rotate the same patient's head 90° to either side.
   NOTE: any movement beyond the anatomical barrier will cause ligament, tendon, or skeletal injury.

   c. In somatic dysfunction, a joint will have **a restrictive (or pathologic) barrier** (see Figure 1.1b). A restrictive barrier lies before the physiologic barrier, and prevents full range of motion of that joint. For example, a patient may have a full range of motion for rotation of the neck to the right. However, the patient may only be able to turn his head to the left approximately 70°. Therefore, a restrictive barrier is met when turning the head to the left.

Trigger Point

Know the difference between physiologic, anatomic and restrictive barriers

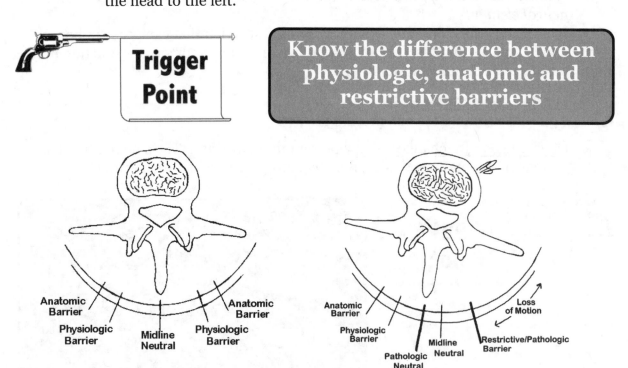

Fig 1.1a: *In a vertebral segment without somatic dysfunction, the vertebrae may rotate equally to either side.* **Fig 1.1b:** *If somatic dysfunction is present, the vertebral segment will not lie in the midline position, and the patient will not be able to rotate the vertebral segment past the restrictive (or pathologic) barrier.*

4. <u>Tenderness</u> - A painful sensation may be produced during palpation of tissues where it should not occur if there were no somatic dysfunction. This is the only subjective component of TART.

C. **Differences between acute and chronic somatic dysfunction**

TART findings will be altered as an injury changes from acute to chronic.

Table 1.1 describes findings in acute vs. chronic somatic dysfunction. [1 p.405, 2 p.17]

Table 1.1

Findings	Acute	Chronic

Tissue texture changes
    Muscle
 	
    Skin
 	
    Soft Tissues
	Increased tone, spasm
	
	Warm, Moist, Red, Inflammed
	
	Boggy, edematous, fluid bulid up from vascular leakage
		Decreased tone, flaccid, mushy
		
		Cool, pale
		
		Doughy, stringy, fibrotic, thickened, contracted

Asymmetry	Present	Present with compensation in other areas of the body.
Restriction	Present, painful with movement	Present, decreased or no pain.
Tenderness	Greatest	Present but less
Viscero-somatic relexes	Uncommon or minimal	Common

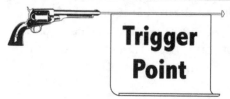

Trigger Point

Know the findings regarding acute vs. chronic somatic dysfunction.

II. **Fryette's Laws**

A. <u>Law I</u>

In 1918, Harrison Fryette noted, with the use of the Halladay spine, that there were certain rules to spinal motion in the thoracic and lumbar regions. Fryette combined the principles of somatic dysfunction and these rules to establish what are now regarded as Fryette's laws. Fryette's laws act as guidelines for physicians to discriminate between different types of dysfunctions, and to determine diagnoses.

Fryette noticed that *if the spine is in the neutral position (no flexion or extension), and if sidebending is introduced, rotation would then occur to the opposite side (Figure 1.2).* This typically applies to more than two vertebral segments (i.e. a group of vertebrae). For example, if a person were to sidebend at T6 - L2, the bodies of the vertebrae would rotate in the opposite direction. He noticed that if a group of vertebrae is in the neutral position and was restricted in left rotation, then the group of vertebrae is rotated right and sidebent left.

Summary of Law I (Figure 1.2)
> In the neutral position:
> *sidebending precedes rotation,*
> *sidebending and rotation occur to*
>   *opposite sides.*

Fryette used this principle for nomenclature of somatic dysfunction:

> e.g.: $NS_L R_R$ = neutral, sidebent left, rotated right.

> **MEMORY TOOL:**
>
> **"N" for Neutral**, the arrows point in the opposite directions, therefore sidebending and rotation are in opposite directions.

B. Law II

Fryette noticed that if *the spine is in the nonneutral position (either flexed nor extended), and rotation is introduced, sidebending would then occur to the same side (Figure 1.3).* This typically applies to a single vertebral segment. For example, if a person were to rotate to the left in the flexed or extended position at the lumbar spine, one vertebral segment would rotate and sidebend in the same direction. He applied this rule to somatic dysfunction, and noticed if L2 is either flexed or extended and restricted in left rotation, then L2 is rotated right and sidebent right. This became Fryette's second law of spinal motion.

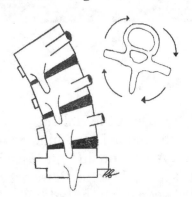

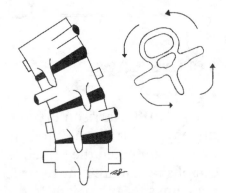

Fig. 1.2: *Fryette's Law I: Left side bending without flexion or extension will cause right rotation of all vertebrae.*

Fig. 1.3: *Fryette's Law II: Left sidebending with flexion or extension will cause one vertebra to rotate to the same side*

MEMORY TOOL:

In "**F**"lexed or
"**E**"xtended lesions,
the arrows point
in the same direction
Therefore,
rotation and
sidebending
are in the same
direction.

Summary of Law II (Figure 1.3)
In a non-neutral (flexed or extended) position: *rotation precedes sidebending, sidebending and rotation occur to the same side.*

Fryette used this principle for nomenclature of somatic dysfunction:
    e.g.: FR_RS_R or FRS_R = flexed, rotated and sidebent right.

**Law I is typical of group dysfunctions.
    For example: L2-L5 NS_RR_L or NSR_L.

**Law II is typical of a single vertebral dysfunction.
    For example: T5 FR_RS_R or FRS_R.

C. **Law III:**
    This was proposed by C.R. Nelson in 1948. He stated that initiating motion at any vertebral segment in any one plane of motion will modify the mobility of that segment in the other two planes of motion. [1 p.432] For example, forward bending will decrease the ability to sidebend and rotate.

NOTE:

Fryette's laws I and II only apply to the thoracic and lumbar vertebrae, NOT the cervical vertebrae!

III. <u>Naming and evaluating somatic dysfunctions</u>

A. <u>Naming somatic dysfunctions</u>

As mentioned above, somatic dysfunction is diagnosed by **TART** (tenderness, asymmetry, restriction, and tissue texture changes). When evaluating somatic dysfunction the physician will examine all of these components, especially restriction. Evaluation of restriction will allow the physician to diagnose and name the somatic dysfunction.

In the case of vertebral segments, motion will occur in flexion/extension, rotation, and sidebending to either side. Therefore, restriction can occur in any of these three planes. When referring to segmental motion, or restriction, *it is traditional to refer to excessive motion (or restriction) of the vertebra **above** in a functional vertebral unit (two vertebrae).* For example, when describing the excessive motion (or restriction) of L2, it is this motion (or restriction) of L2 on L3.

Somatic dysfunctions of the spine are always named for their freedom of motion.

Three examples of nomenclature:

1. If L2 is restricted in the motions of flexion, sidebending to the right and rotation to the right, then L2 is said to be extended, rotated and sidebent to the left on L3. This is denoted as L2 ER_LS_L or ERS_L.
2. If T5 is restricted in the motions of extension, sidebending to the left and rotating to the left, then T5 is said to be flexed, rotated and sidebent to the right on T6. This is denoted as T5 FR_RSR or FRS_R.
3. If T5 - T10 is not restricted in flexion or extension, but is restricted in sidebending to the left and rotating to the right, then T5 is said to be neutral, sidebent right and rotated left. The nomenclature is denoted as T5 - T10 NS_RR_L.

B. <u>Evaluating somatic dysfunctions</u>

Cervical spine
See Chapter 2 Cervical Spine section II D "Motion testing."

Thoracic and lumbar spine

1. **Assess rotation by placing the thumbs over the transverse processes (TP's) of each segment.**
   If the right thumb is more posterior than the left thumb, then the segment is rotated right.

2. **Check the rotation of the segment in flexion.**
   If the rotation gets better (i.e. the right thumb is no longer posterior), this suggests that the segment is flexed, sidebent and rotated right FR_RS_R.

3. **Check the segment in extension.**
   If the rotation gets better in extension, this suggests that the segment is extended, sidebent and rotated right ER_RS_R.

If the rotation remains the same in flexion and extension, then the segments are neutral sidebent left and rotated right $NSLR_R$.

Algorithm for evaluating somatic dysfunction

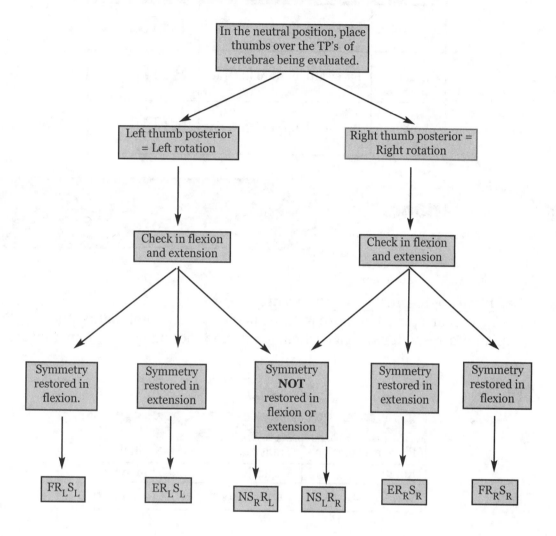

VI. <u>Facet orientation and spinal motion</u>

A. <u>Orientation of SUPERIOR facets</u>
Facet orientation will determine the motion of the vertebral segments. For example, if a pair of facets were to face backward and medial, then sagittal plane motion would be favored (flexion and extension). An easy mnemonic to remember the orientation of superior facets in the axial skeleton is shown in Table 1.2.

Table 1.2

Region	Facet Orientation	Mnemonic
Cervical	Backward, upward, medial	**BUM**
Thoracic	Backward, upward, lateral	**BUL**
Lumbar	Backward, upward, medial	**BUM**

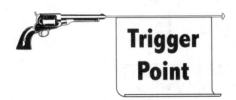

Trigger Point

Know the superior facets' orientations.

B. Physiologic motion of the spine
The human spine can move in three planes or any combination thereof. Each plane corresponds with a particular axis and motion as shown in Table 1.3.

Table 1.3

Motion	Axis	Plane
Flexion/extension	Transverse	Sagittal
Rotation	Vertical	Transverse
Sidebending	Anterior - posterior	Coronal

V. Muscle contraction

A. Isotonic contraction – Muscle contraction that results in the approximation of the muscle's origin and insertion without a change in its tension. In such a case the operator's force is less than the patient's force. [1 p.1090]

B. Isometric contraction – Muscle contraction that results in the increase in tension without an approximation of origin and insertion. In such a case the operator's force and the patient's force are equal. [1 p.1090]

C. Isolytic contraction – Muscle contraction against resistance *while forcing* the muscle to lengthen. In such a case the operator's force is more than the patient's force. [1 p.1090]

D. Concentric contraction – Muscle contraction that results in the approximation of the muscle's origin and insertion. [1 p.1090]

E. **Eccentric contraction** – Lengthening of muscle during contraction due to an external force. [1 p.1090]

VI. Osteopathic Treatment

A. Direct vs. Indirect Treatment

As mentioned earlier, all somatic dysfunctions will have a restrictive (pathologic) barrier. This restrictive barrier will inhibit movement in one direction thus causing asymmetry within the joint or tissue. The goal of osteopathic treatment is to eliminate this restrictive barrier, thus restoring symmetry.

Osteopathic practitioners use a variety of treatments to achieve this goal. All of these treatments fall into two categories, **direct treatment** and **indirect treatment.**

In a *direct treatment*, the practitioner "engages" the restrictive barrier. This means that the body tissues and/or joints are eventually moved *through* the restrictive barrier. This can be done by direct palpation of the dysfunctional tissues or using a body part as a lever.

For example:

1. If T3 was FR_RS_R, the practitioner would extend, rotate and sidebend T3 to the left.
2. If the abdominal fascia moved more freely cephalad than caudad, the practitioner would hold the tissue caudad (toward the barrier), allowing the tissues to stretch.

In an *indirect treatment* the practitioner moves tissues and/or joints *away from* the restrictive barrier into the direction of freedom.

For example:

1. If T3 was FR_RS_R, the practitioner would flex, sidebend and rotate T3 to the right.
2. If the abdominal fascia moved more freely cephalad than caudad, the practitioner would hold the tissue cephalad (away from the barrier) allowing the tissues to relax.

B. Passive vs. Active Treatment

In an active treatment, the patient will assist in the treatment, usually in the form of isometric or isotonic contraction.

In a passive treatment, the patient will relax and allow the practitioner to move the body tissues.

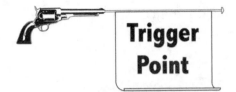

Direct Treatment ———→ Towards the barrier

Indirect Treatment ——→ Away from
the barrier

Active Treatment ———→ Patient assists
during treatment.

Passive Treatment ———→ Patient relaxes
during treatment.

Table 1.4

Treatment Type	Direct or Indirect	Active or Passive
Myofascial Release	Both	Both
Counterstrain	Indirect	Passive
Facilitated Positional Release	Indirect	Passive
Osteopathy in the Cranial Field	Both	Passive
Lymphatic treatment	Direct	Passive
Chapman's reflexes	Direct	Passive

VII. Treatment Plan

A. Choice of Treatment
Precise answers to choice of technique do not exist; there are only general guidelines. [3 p.576-7]

1. Elderly patients and hospitalized patients typically respond better to indirect techniques or gentle direct techniques such as articulatory techniques.
2. The use of HVLA in a patient with advanced osteoporosis or metastatic cancer may lead to a pathologic fracture. [3 p.576-7]
3. Acute neck strain/sprains are often better treated with indirect techniques to prevent further strain.

B. Dose and Frequency
Absolute rules for dose and frequency do not exist. Typical guidelines are as follows: [3 p.576-7]

1. For sicker patients, limit the OMT to a few key areas.
2. Allow time for the patient's body to respond to the treatment that was given.
3. Pediatric patients can be treated more frequently, whereas geriatric patients may need a longer time to respond to the treatment.
4. Acute cases should have a shorter interval between treatments; as they respond to the treatment, the interval can be increased.

C. Sequencing of Treatment
There are different opinions regarding what should be treated first. Guidelines on sequencing are not absolute. Each physician after gaining experience develops his or her own approach.

The following is a sample sequence: [3 p.576-7]

1. For psoas syndrome, treat the lumbar spine [3 p.577] or thoraco-lumbar spine[4] first.
2. Treat the ribs and upper thoracic spine before treating the cervical spine.
3. Treat the thoracic spine before treating rib dysfunctions.
4. For acute somatic dysfunctions, treating peripheral areas will allow access to the acute area.
5. Cranial treatment can make the patient relax. This will allow OMT to work in other areas.
6. For extremity problems, treat the spine, sacrum and ribs first (axial skeleton).

Chapter 1 Review Questions

1. A 50-year-old male with no history of low back pain presents with acute low back pain after gardening for several hours yesterday. Structural examination reveals tissue texture changes to the right lumbar paraspinal region. Which of the following would most likely be appreciated at this time?

   A. cool dry skin
   B. hypertonicity
   C. fibrosis
   D. itching
   E. paresthesia

2. A 60-year-old female presents for a general wellness examination. She denies any complaints and has no noticeable limitations to range of motion by routine musculoskeletal examination. However, focused osteopathic structural examination reveals somatic dysfunction of T1-T2 on the left, and fibrotic muscles with decreased tension. Which of the following is most associated with this type of somatic dysfunction?

   A. cool dry skin
   B. articular motion restrictions and sharp pain with movement
   C. segmental asymmetry without noticeable compensation in other areas of the body
   D. erythema
   E. moist, edematous, and boggy tissue

3. A 40-year-old presents with mid-thoracic pain of 1 weeks duration. Structural examination reveals that T6 is ER_LS_L. Which of the following is most associated with this segment's restrictions?
   A. extension, rotation and sidebending to the left in relation to T5
   B. extension, rotation and sidebending to the left in relation to T7
   C. flexion, rotation and sidebending to the left in relation to T7
   D. flexion, rotation and sidebending to the right in relation to T5
   E. flexion, rotation and sidebending to the right in relation to T7

4. A 25-year-old male complains of upper back pain. Structural examination reveals T2 is restricted with left rotation. Flexing the body down to T2 causes the segment to further rotate to the right, while extending the area causes T2 to return to the neutral position. The most appropriate nomenclature for this dysfunction is?

   A. ER_LS_L
   B. ER_RS_R
   C. FR_LS_L
   D. FR_RS_R
   E. NR_RS_L

5. A 75-year-old male has chronic low back pain due to known metastatic prostate cancer to the lumbar vertebrae. The most appropriate osteopathic manipulative therapy is

    A. facilitated positional release to the lumbar spine
    B. high velocity low amplitude to the lumbar spine
    C. Counterstain to the cervical spine
    D. muscle energy to the lumbar spine
    E. pelvic diaphragm release

6. A 40-year-old male with presents with a thoracic curve. History reveals it had a dull achy quality. Structural examination reveals a large paraspinal hump on the left side. Which of the following is the most likely diagnosis?

    A. T4-7 $ER_R S_L$
    B. T5-9 $NR_L S_L$
    C. T6 $NR_L S_L$
    D. T7-9 $NR_L S_R$
    E. T8 $FR_R S_R$

The following refer to questions 7-9:
A 20-year-old female presents for a general maintenance examination without complaints. Structural examination is negative for somatic dysfunction.

7. The patient without a cervical somatic dysfunction actively sidebends her cervical spine to an endpoint of 45 degrees. This limit is most appropriately described as the

    A. anatomic barrier
    B. elastic barrier
    C. physiologic barrier
    D. restrictive barrier
    E. rotational barrier

8. The examiner evaluates the physiologic motion of T3 on T4. Which of the following most accurately describes this segment's Fryette Type 2 mechanics?

    A. Initiating motion of the segment in any plane of motion will modify the movement of that segment in other planes of motion
    B. When the spine is in a neutral position, the coupled motions of sidebending and rotation occur in opposite directions with rotation occurring toward the convexity.
    C. When the spine is in a neutral position, the coupled motions of sidebending and rotation occur in the same direction
    D. When the spine is sufficiently forward or backward bent, the coupled motions of sidebending and rotation occur in opposite directions with rotation occurring toward the convexity
    E. When the spine is sufficiently forward or backward bent, the coupled motions of sidebending and rotation occur in the same direction.

9. The orientation of the superior facets in the thoracic spine is best described as

> A. backward and medial
> B. backward, upward, and lateral
> C. backward, upward, and medial
> D. forward and medial
> E. forward, upward, and lateral

The following refer to questions 10 and 11:

> For each numbered item (description) select one heading (physiologic motion) most closely associated with it. Each lettered heading may be selected once, more than once, or not at all.

> A. flexion and extension
> B. neutral
> C. rotation
> D. rotation and sidebending
> E. sidebending

10. Normal motion of the vertebral segments in a sagittal plane

> A. A
> B. B
> C. C
> D. D
> E. E

11. Motion of vertebral segments around a vertical axis

> A. A
> B. B
> C. C
> D. D
> E. E

The following refer to questions 12-15:

> For each numbered item (description) select one heading (muscle contraction) most closely associated with it. Each lettered heading may be selected once, more than once, or not at all.

> A. concentric
> B. eccentric
> C. isolytic
> D. isometric
> E. isotonic

12. The activity of the biceps muscle during the elevation of a weight while performing a curling maneuver is indicative of

    A. A
    B. B
    C. C
    D. D
    E. E

13. The activity of the biceps muscle while holding a weight steady with arms flexed at 90 degrees

    A. A
    B. B
    C. C
    D. D
    E. E

14. The activity of the biceps muscle while lowering a weight during a curling exercise

    A. A
    B. B
    C. C
    D. D
    E. E

15. Muscle contraction against resistance while and external force causes the muscle to lengthen with the purpose of breaking adhesions

    A. A
    B. B
    C. C
    D. D
    E. E

Explanations

1. Answer: **B**

    This patient has an acute somatic dysfunction. These are characterized in early stages by boggy edema, tenderness, and pain. Acute somatic dysfunctions are also associated with increased temperature and moisture, erythema, and hypertonic musculature.

2. Answer: **A**

    This patient has a chronic somatic dysfunction. These are characterized by dull and achy tenderness, cool and dry skin with slight tension, and decreased muscular tension. Also the skin may be thickened, and/or contracted with a rapidly fading red reflex upon blanching. [3 p. 1118]

3. Answer: **E**

    Vertebral segments are always described in relation to the vertebrae below. In this example, T6 motion is described in relation to T7. Somatic dysfunctions are named for the freedom of motion. Thus T6 is at ease in extension and left-sided rotation and sidebending. Therefore, it is restricted in flexion, rotation and sidebending to the right.

4. Answer: **B**

    Somatic dysfunction is named for the freedom of motion. Therefore, the T2 segment is rotated right and is restricted in left rotation. The segment is also more free with extension as it is described returning more to neutral position with this motion. Thus, T2 is now known to be extended and rotated right. Since only T2 demonstrates non-neutral mechanics (flexed or extended) it follows Fryette type II mechanics where the segment sidebends and rotates in the same direction. Therefore since the segment is rotated right it must sidebent right.

5. Answer: **A**

    There are several relative contraindications to OMT. Performing HVLA or muscle energy (both direct techniques) on someone with active boney metastases can theoretically cause a pathologic fracture. Lymphatic techniques can hasten metastasis by augmenting the autonomic and lymphatic systems of the involved regions. Thus, the most indirect therapy listed is the most appropriate treatment modality in this situation. Counterstain to the cervical spine alone would not be the most appropriate treatment for someone with low back pain.

6. Answer: **D**

Group curves typically follow Fryette type I mechanics where the segments are in the neutral position and sidebend and rotate to the same side. Group curves can be associated with chronic somatic dysfunctions such that they have a dull, achy character. In this question, the patient has a left paraspinal hump (the paraspinals on the left are more prominent posteriorly). Therefore, the segments are rotated to the left. Since it is neutral, rotated left, it must be sidebent right. Of note, a single (non-neutral) somatic dysfunction will not usually cause a large paraspinal hump.

7. Answer: **C**

This patient has no pathologic/restrictive barriers due to having a negative osteopathic structural examination for restrictions or asymmetry. The physiologic barrier is the limit of active (patient-mediated) motion. The anatomic barrier is the limit of passive (physician-mediated) motion. The elastic barrier is a range between these two in which passive ligamentous stretching occurs before tissue disruption.

8. Answer: **E**

Thoracic or lumbar somatic dysfunctions follow Fryette type II mechanics in which a single vertebral unit will sidebend and rotate in the same direction when the vertebra is significantly flexed or extended. Rotation occurs into the concavity of the curve.

9. Answer: **B**

The thoracic facets are oriented 60 degrees from the transverse plane and 20 degrees from the frontal plane to allow lateral bending, rotation, and some flexion and extension. They are oriented backward, upward, and lateral. The lumbar and cervical facets are oriented backward, upward and medial.

10. Answer: **A**

The sagittal plane passes longitudinally through the body from front to back, dividing it into right and left portions. Extension or flexion is the accepted universal term for backward or forward motion of the spine, respectively, in the sagittal plane about a transverse axis. Neutral positioning is better described as the range of sagittal plane spinal positioning in which the first principle of physiologic motion of the spine applies.

11. Answer: **C**

The vertical (longitudinal) axis is formed by the intersection of the sagittal and coronal planes, which is a midpoint on the anterior-superior surface of the vertebral body. Rotation occurs about this axis. Sidebending occurs in a coronal (frontal) plane about an anterior-posterior axis.

12. Answer: **A**

Concentric contraction is the normal muscle action we think of when actively lifting weights. It results in approximation of the muscle attachments during contraction. As the weight swings through an arc while curling, the tension of the muscle is variable.

13. Answer: **D**

An example of an isometric contraction would be carrying an object in front of you. The weight of the object would be pulling downward, but your hands and arms would be opposing the motion with equal force going upwards.

14. Answer: **B**

Eccentric contraction is the lengthening of a muscle during a contraction due to an external force. As the weight is dropped down from the curled position the biceps is contracting while the muscle is lengthening.

15. Answer: **C**

Isolytic contractions are a type of eccentric contraction designed to break adhesions using an operator-induced force to lengthen the muscle against resistance. The counterforce is greater than the patient force.

Cervical Spine 2

I. Anatomy

A. Bones

The cervical spine consists of seven vertebral segments (see fig 2.1). C1 and C2 are considered atypical. C1 has no spinous process or vertebral body. C2 has a dens that projects superiorly from its body and articulates with C1. C2 – C6 generally have bifid spinous processes. The articular pillars (or lateral masses) are the portion of bone of the cervical vertebral segments that lie between the superior and inferior facets. The articular pillars are located posterior to the cervical transverse processes, and are used by osteopathic physicians to evaluate cervical vertebral motion. Foramen transversarium are foramina in the transverse process of C1-C6 that allow for the passage of the vertebral artery.

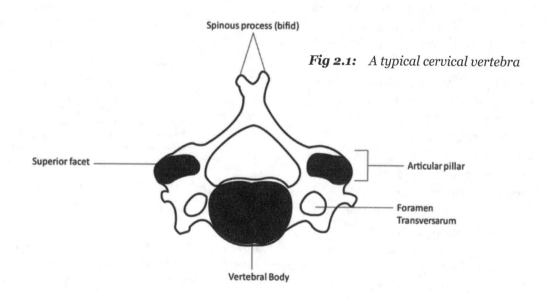

Spinous process (bifid)

Fig 2.1: *A typical cervical vertebra*

Superior facet

Articular pillar

Foramen Transversarium

Vertebral Body

B. Muscles

Scalenes (anterior, middle, posterior) - Originate from the posterior tubercle of the transverse processes of the cervical vertebrae and insert onto rib 1 (anterior and middle) and rib 2 (posterior). [5 p.783] They sidebend the neck to the same side with unilateral contraction, and flex the neck with bilateral contraction. The scalenes also aid in respiration. *The anterior and middle scalene will help elevate the first rib during forced inhalation. The posterior scalene will help elevate the second rib during forced inhalation.* [5 p.793] It is common to have a tender point in one of the scalenes (posterior to the clavicle at the base of the neck) with a first or second inhalation rib dysfunction.

Sternocleidomastoid (SCM) - Originates from the mastoid process and the lateral half of the superior nuchal line. Inserts onto the medial 1/3 of the clavicle and sternum. With unilateral contraction, the SCM will sidebend ipsilaterally and rotate contralaterally (sidebend toward and rotate away). Bilateral contraction will flex the neck. *The SCM divides the neck into anterior and posterior triangles.* [5 p.786] Shortening or restrictions within the SCM often results in torticollis.

C. Ligaments

The *alar* ligament extends from the sides of the dens to the lateral margins of the foramen magnum. The *transverse* ligament of the atlas attaches to the lateral masses of C1 to hold the dens in place. Rheumatoid arthritis and Down Syndrome can weaken these ligaments leading to atlanto-axial subluxation. Rupture of this ligament (which may occur with rheumatoid arthritis and Down Syndrome) will result in catastrophic neurological damage. [1 p.515]

D. Joints

Joints of Luschka – The uncinate processes are superior lateral projections originating from the posterior lateral rim of the vertebral bodies of C3 - C7. [6 p.79] They help support the lateral side of the cervical discs and protect cervical nerve roots from disc herniation. [7 p. 210, 6 p.79] *The articulation of the superior uncinate process and the superadjacent vertebra is known as the Joint of Luschka.* [6 p.373] These joints have also been called uncovertebral joints. [6 p.5] They may or may not be considered true synovial joints, but play an important role in cervical motion, especially

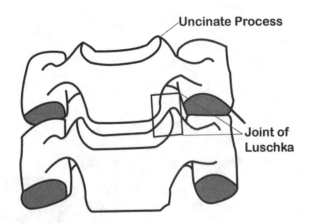

Fig 2.2: *Joints of Luschka (also known as uncovertebral joints). Formed by the articulation of the uncinate process and the superadjacent vertebra.*

sidebending. [7 p.210] *Since the Joints of Luschka are in close proximity to the intervertebral foramina, degenerative changes and hypertrophy can lead to foraminal stenosis and nerve root compression.* [7 p.212] The most common cause of cervical nerve root pressure is degeneration of the Joints of Luschka in addition to hypertrophic arthritis of the intervertebral synovial (facet) joints. [7 p.214]

E   Nerves
There are 8 cervical nerve roots (see fig 2.3). *The upper seven exit above their corresponding vertebra.* For example, the C7 nerve root will exit between C6 and C7. The last cervical nerve root (C8) will exit between C7 and T1. The brachial plexus is made up of nerve roots from C5 - T1. Therefore, damage to the lower cervical cord will cause neurological symptoms in the upper extremity.

> **NOTE:**
>
> **Fryette's laws I and II only apply to the thoracic and lumbar vertebrae, NOT the cervical vertebrae.**

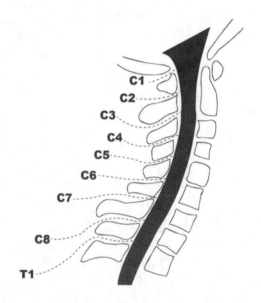

Fig 2.3:   *Nerve roots in the cervical region will exit above the corresponding vertebra.*

II. **Motion and mechanics**

A. **Occipital-atlantal (OA) motion** – The OA is considered to be the motion of the occipital condyles on the atlas (C1). *Its primary motion is flexion and extension.* Approximately 50% of the flexion and extension of the cervical spine stems from the OA joint. [7 p.188] *Sidebending and rotation occur to opposite sides with either flexion or extension.* Therefore, if the OA is flexed, sidebent left and rotated right, then this means that the occiput on the atlas is flexed, sidebent left and rotated right (FR_RS_L).

B. <u>Atlantal-axial (AA) motion</u> – The AA is considered to be C1 motion on C2. *Its primary motion is rotation (50% of the rotation of the cervical spine occurs here [7 p.189, 1 p.518]). Clinically only rotation occurs at this joint.* [7 p.208] Therefore, if the AA is rotated right this means that the atlas (C1) is rotated right on the axis (C2). Although cineradiographic studies show a significant amount of flexion and extension occuring at the atlas, this motion does not seem to be involved in somatic dysfunction. [1 p.518]

C. <u>Inferior division (C2-C7)</u> – It is generally accepted that *sidebending and*

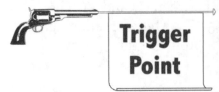

Segment	Main Motion	Sidebending and rotation
OA	Flexion and Extension	Opposite Sides
AA	Rotation	
C2-C4	Rotation	Same Sides
C5-C7	Sidebending	Same Sides

rotation occur to the same side. However, some authors believe that the C7/T1 facet joint is more thoracic in configuration and thus tends to follow Fryette mechanics. [1 p.433] The inferior division accounts for 50% of the flexion/extension and 50% of the rotation of the entire cervical spine. [7 p.189]

D. <u>Motion testing</u>
1. **<u>Occipital-atlantal (OA) motion testing</u>** – [1 p.521, 7 p.579 - 581]
   Translation – Cup the occiput with both hands, with the finger tips and middle finger over the occipito-atlantal articulation. Move the occiput on the atlas by translating to the left then the right. Lateral translation of the occiput to the right (right translation) will produce left sidebending. Therefore, if the OA is restricted in right translation in the flexed position, this suggests an occiput that is extended, rotated left and sidebent right (i.e., restriction of flexion, rotating right and sidebending left).

   Right Translation = Force from Left to Right = Left Sidebending

   Rotation – To detect occipital rotation, stabilize the arch of the atlas with the thumb and index finger. The other hand is placed on top of the skull and rotate to the right and left evaluating freedom and resistance. [7 p.580]

   Sidebending – Place finger pads in the occipital sulci and determine the depth of each sulci. Left occipital sidebending will seperate the right occipital condyle and atlas; as a result the right sulcus will feel deep. Since sidebending and rotation are toward opposite sides, a right deep sulcus indicates left sidebending, which indicates right rotation.

Somatic dysfunction –
In the above example where the OA is rotated left and sidebent right, the occiput will feel more posteror on the left. If there is tenderness and tissue texture abnormalities on the left, it is called a **posterior occiput left**. If the tenderness and tissue texture abnormalities are on the right, it is called an **anterior occiput right**.[1 p.521]

2. **Atlantal-axial (AA) motion testing** – [1 p.521-5, 7 p.582-3,]
   Rotation – Grasp the head with the finger tips contacting the lateral mass of the atlas. Flex the neck to 45° and rotate the head to the right and left. Flexing the cervical spine to 45° will lock out rotation of the typical cervical vertebrae (C2 - C7). A right rotated atlas exhibits restriction in left rotation, and vice versa.

   Somatic dysfunction – [1 p.521]
   If the atlas is rotated to the left, the atlas will feel more posteror on the left. If there is tenderness and tissure texture abnormalities on the left it is called a **posterior atlas left**. If the same rotation is true in the above example (rotated left) however, the tenderness and tissue texture abnormalities are on the right it is called an **anterior atlas right**. Anterior atlas dysfunctions are uncommon and associated with retroorbital pain. [1 p.521]

3. **C2-C7 motion testing** – [1 p.521]
   Translation - The translation test is similar to the occiput translation test, except that the physician's finger tips placed over the lateral border of the articular pillars. Lateral translation of the cervical spine to the right (right translation) will produce left sidebending. Therefore, if C3 is restricted in right translation in the flexed position, it suggests that C3 is extended, rotated right and sidebent right.

   Rotation –
   Method # 1: With the patient's head supported, place the finger tips of the index finger on the posterior surface of the articular pillars. Rotate to the right and left evaluating freedom or resistance.
   Method # 2: With the patient's head supported, contact the posterior aspect of the lateral mass with the index finger tips. Push directly anterior with the right finger to induce left rotation, then do the same with the left finger to induce right rotation.[7 p.582]

III.   Important considerations about the cervical spine

Suboccipital or paravertebral muscle spasms are usually associated with upper thoracic or rib problems on the same side. Therefore, treat these areas first, then treat the cervical spine. [1 p.525]

An acute injury to the cervical spine is best treated with indirect fascial techniques or counterstrain first. [1 p.525]

Cervical foraminal stenosis [7 p.212, 219-20]

Definition – Degenerative changes within the joints of Luschka, hypertrophic changes of the intervertebral (facet) joints, and osteophyte formation associated with arthritis, may result in intervertebral foraminal narrowing. *Degenerative changes within the joints of Luschka along with hypertrophy of the intervertebral (facet) joints is the most common cause of cervical nerve root pressure symptoms.* [7 p.211]

Location of pain – Neck pain radiating into the upper extremity

Quality of pain – Dull ache, shooting pain or paresthesias

Signs and Symptoms – Increased pain with neck extension, positive Spurling's test (see Chapter 18 – Special tests), paraspinal muscle spasm, posterior and anterior cervical tenderpoints

Radiology – Osteophyte formation and degenerative joint changes on AP and lateral views. Oblique views demonstrate narrowing of the intervertebral foramina.

Treatment – OMT should be directed at maintaining optimal range of motion of the cervical spine. Articulatory techniques as well as muscle energy can improve segmental range of motion. Myofacial release, counterstrain, and facilitated positional release can improve myofacial restrictions.

Chapter 2 Review Questions

1. An 18-year-old male presents with right-sided chest pain after a coughing fit. Structural examination reveals a rib exhalation dysfunction on the right side at the Angle of Louis. Which of the following muscles help elevate this rib with forced inhalation?

    A. anterior scalene
    B. middle scalene
    C. pectoralis minor
    D. posterior scalene
    E. sternocleidomastoid

2. A 30-year-old presents with radicular neck pain into the right arm. Physical examination reveals weakness of the deltoid musculature with 4/5 muscle strength to shoulder abduction and external rotation. MRI reveals moderate stenosis of the intervertebral foramen between C2 and C3 as well as C4 and C5. The most likely nerve root affected is

    A. C2
    B. C3
    C. C4
    D. C5
    E. C6

3. A 35-year-old female presents with upper neck pain after a motor vehicle accident. History reveals she was rear-ended as the restrained driver. Structural examination reveals somatic dysfunction of the occiput on the atlas. The most likely somatic dysfunction

    A. is most commonly seen as a flexion restriction with rotation and sidebending restricted to the same side
    B. follows Fryette's principles
    C. occurs typically as sidebending and rotation restrictions
    D. occurs typically as flexion and extension restrictions
    E. occurs as purely a rotational restriction

4. In evaluating a patient with suboccipital pain you find that the atlantoaxial joint is restricted in right rotation. Which of the following statements is most associated with this somatic dysfunction?

    A. C1 on C2 will be restricted in right sidebending
    B. C2 on C3 will be restricted in right sidebending
    C. C1 on C2 will move freely in left rotation
    D. the atlantoaxial joint will typically have associated flexion or extension restrictions
    E. the occiput on C1 will be restricted in right sidebending

5. A 42-year-old female presents with neck pain after a motor vehicle collision. History reveals her car was hit on the passenger side. Motion testing of the occipitoatlantal joint reveals it translates easier to the right. Findings improve in extension. The most likely diagnosis at the occipitoatlantal joint is

    A. extended, rotated left, sidebent left
    B. extended, rotated right, sidebent left
    C. extended, rotated right, sidebent right
    D. flexed, rotated left, sidebent left
    E. flexed, rotated right, sidebent left

6. While diagnosing your patient's neck, you notice that C5 is freer in left rotation. Rotation improves with flexion and becomes restricted in extension. The most likely diagnosis is

    A. flexed, rotated left, sidebent left
    B. flexed, rotated left, sidebent right
    C. flexed, rotated right, sidebent right
    D. extended, rotated left, sidebent left
    E. extended, rotated right, sidebent right

7. In the absence of specifically localizing flexion or extension, when sidebending is introduced to a group of typical cervical vertebrae, the anticipated rotation

    A. does not occur
    B. will occur, but not in a predictable fashion
    C. will occur in the direction of the convexity produced by the sidebending
    D. will occur in the opposite direction to which sidebending has occurred
    E. will occur in the same direction to which sidebending has occurred

8. A neonate presents with parental concern for torticollis. Physical examination reveals spastic contraction of the left sternocleidomastoid muscle. This will cause the cervical spine to

    A. laterally translate right and rotate right
    B. sidebend left and rotate left
    C. sidebend left and rotate right
    D. sidebend right and rotate left
    E. sidebend right and rotate right

9. A 75-year-old male presents with neck pain. Physical examination reveals dizziness when his head is passively rotated and extended. Radiographs reveal moderate degenerative changes of the cervical spine. Compression of which of the following structures is the most likely cause of this patient's symptoms?

    A. brachiocephalic vein
    B. cervical ganglia of sympathetic trunk
    C. nucleus pulposus of the C3-C4 disk
    D. vertebral artery
    E. zygapophyseal joint

10. A 25-year-old male presents with neck pain and requests osteopathic manipulation. A history of which of the following would be most contraindicated to performing HVLA in this patient?

    A. Down syndrome
    B. fibromyalgia
    C. herniated cervical disc
    D. osteoarthritis
    E. quadriparesis

Questions 11-13 refer to the following:

    A 20-year-old female presents for a general maintenance examination without complaints. A comprehensive musculoskeletal examination is unremarkable. Structural examination is reveals a slight tissue texture change in the cervical region.

11. Which of the following is most consistent with the physiologic mechanics of this patient's cervical spine?

    A. decreased translation to the right at C4 suggests that C4 is restricted in left sidebending
    B. the C2/C3 vertebral unit is responsible for more than 50% of the overall rotation of the cervical spine
    C. the primary motion of the lower cervical spine is flexion and extension
    D. the primary motion of the lower cervical spine is rotation
    E. the uncinate process of the cervical spine is located on the spinous process

12. The physician palpates the articular masses on the lateral aspect of her cervical vertebrae. These are most appropriately described as

    A. anterior to the cervical transverse processes
    B. cervical transverse processes
    C. the bone located between the superior and inferior facets
    D. medial to the cervical lamina
    E. medial to the cervical pedicle

13. The physician then flexes the neck to 45 degrees and rotates the head. Which of the following vertebrae is best assessed with this approach?

   A. OA
   B. C1
   C. C2
   D. C3
   E. C4

Questions 14-15 refer to the following:

For each numbered item (patient presentation) select one heading (somatic dysfunction) most closely associated with it. Each lettered heading may be selected once, more than once, or not at all.

   A. rotated left
   B. rotated right
   C. sidebent left
   D. extended
   E. flexed

14. A 65-year-old male with chronic headaches has an occipitoatlantal joint restricted in right translation. The most likely somatic dysfunction for the affected region is

   A. A
   B. B
   C. C
   D. D
   E. E

15. A 45-year-old truck driver has difficulty looking over his left shoulder to check his blind spot. The most likely somatic dysfunction of the atlas is

   A. A
   B. B
   C. C
   D. D
   E. E

Explanations

1. Answer: **D**

    The Angle of Louis is the anatomic landmark for the sternal angle and attaches to the 2nd rib (see Chapter 3 . The posterior scalene attaches to the second rib and can help to elevate this exhalation dysfunction of rib 2 with forced inhalation. Refer to the chapter on ribs for more information on treatment of rib dysfunctions.

2. Answer: **D**

    It is pertinent to review basic muscle actions and their associated neuromusculoskeletal exam findings (see appendix B in this text) prior to test day. This patient has findings consistent with stenosis of the C5 root which is located above the C5 vertebra at the C4/5 foramen. C5 partially innervated the deltoid (shoulder abduction) and infraspinatus (external rotation). Note that the cervical spinal cord segments exit above the level of their associated vertebrae with the C8 root exiting above the level of the first thoracic vertebrae. Although the patient has stenosis at C3/4, the C3 nerve root would be affected however this would not result in any arm weakness since the brachial plexus begings with the C5 nerve root. C3 is primarily responsible for innervating the cervical paraspinals

3. Answer: **D**

    The main motion of the occipitoatlantal joint is flexion and extension with a small amount of rotation and sidebending. While the OA does in fact typically rotate and sidebend in opposite directions, the main restriction will be in alignment with the segment's main motions of flexion and extension – especially given the patient's mechanism of injury.

4. Answer: **C**

    Vertebral segments with somatic dysfunction are always described in relation to the vertebrae below the described area. The atlantoaxial joint is C1-C2 and primarily moves in rotation. Clinically, only rotation occurs at this joint. Therefore, if the atlantoaxial joint is restricted in right rotation, it will move more freely in left rotation. Sidebending is not considered a significant component of atlas movement. [1 p.518] Although flexion and extension occurs at this joint, these motions are not typically involved with somatic dysfunction [1 p.518]

5. Answer: **B**

Somatic dysfunction is named for the freedom of motion. This patient has an OA that moves free with right translation (i.e. left sidebending). Findings improve in extension, therefore the OA is extended sidebent left. Since the OA is known to rotate and sidebend in opposite directions, the OA is rotated right. Therefore, the OA is extended, rotated right, and sidebent left.

6. Answer: **A**

Somatic dysfunction is named for the freedom of motion. Since motion is freer with left rotation it is considered rotated left. Since C5 rotates and sidebands to the same side the segment must be sidebent left as well. If the segment is freer in flexion compared to extension, it is considered flexed. Thus, the segment is flexed, rotated left and sidebent left.

7. Answer: **E**

Typical cervical vertebrae (C2-C7) generally rotate and sidebend in the same directions. They can be flexed, extended, or neutral, but they do not follow Fryette mechanics. Become familiar with the terms convexity and concavity for nomenclature and testing purposes. The direction of convexity is away from the direction of sidebending.

8. Answer: **C**

The sternocleidomastoid muscle connects the mastoid process to the sternum and clavicle in a diagonal fashion. Contraction of this muscle causes sidebending to the affected side and rotation away. Therefore, a left sternocleidomastoid contracture will sidebend the head to the left and rotate it to the right.

9. Answer: **D**

There are several risks involved with performing HVLA and one must understand the regional anatomy to appreciate these risks. Severe neurovascular accidents can be associated with upper cervical manipulation such as vertebral artery compression with thrombosis, occipitobasilar strokes (Wallenberg syndrome), arterial dissections, or cerebellar infarctions. These primarily occur with use of rotational forces with the head extended, thereby compressing or manipulating the vertebral artery within the transverse foramen. They are the most common adverse event of cervical manipulation cited in literature at a rate of 1:400,000 to 1 in 1 million.

10. Answer: **A**

Patients with rheumatoid arthritis and Down syndrome are at risk during direct cervical manipulation because the odontoid ligament can be weakened and susceptible to rupture . (see Chapter 16 HVLA absolute contraindications). Complications, such as fracture are associated with the following underlying conditions: osteoporosis, metastatic bone disease, bone infections, vertebral tuberculosis. Exacerbation of a herniated disc with acute radiculopathy is a possible complication but is cited to be rare in literature compared to the combination of vascular events described above.

11.   Answer: **A**

Right translation = force from left to right = left sidebending. Therefore, if C4 is restricted in right translation it suggests that C4 is restricted in left sidebending. Typical cervical vertebrae (C2-C7) generally flex/extend and sidebend and rotate in the same direction. The lower cervicals are responsible for 50% of overall rotation and sidebending of the cervical spine. The uncinate process is a hook-shaped process on the top surface of the bodies of most cervical vertebrae.

12.   Answer: **C**

The bone between the superior and inferior articular facets which we palpate and consider as a transverse process is known as the articular pillar. The lateral portions of the atlas are known as lateral masses.

13.   Answer: **B**

Flexing the cervical spine to 45 degrees helps to lock rotation for the remainder of the typical cervical vertebrae (C2-C7) and isolate rotation of the atlas (C1).

14.   Answer: **A**

The OA joint rotates and sidebends in opposite directions. This patient has a restriction in right translation which is inducing sidebending to the left. So if the OA is restricted in left sidebending, it is called sidebent right because it has an ease of motion in this direction. It must also be rotated left if following known segmental mechanics of this region. Therefore this patient's OA is sidebent right and rotated left.

15.   Answer: **B**

This patient most likely has a rotated right atlas. The truck driver is having difficulty in turning his head to the left. Therefore his atlas is limited in left rotation. The atlas will then rotate right with ease.

Thorax and Ribcage **3**

Thorax

I. Anatomy

A. Rule of three's

Spinous processes are large and point increasingly downward from T1-T9, then back to almost an anterior-posterior orientation from T10-T12. [8 p.563] A useful way to identify the thoracic transverse processes from the location of the corresponding spinous process involves the **"rule of three's:"**

1. <u>T1-T3</u> - the spinous process is *located at the level of the corresponding transverse process.*
2. <u>T4-T6</u> - the spinous process is *located one-half a segment below the corresponding transverse process.* For example, the spinous process of T5 is located halfway between the tranverse processes of T5 and T6.
3. <u>T7-T9</u> - the spinous process is *located at the level of the transverse process of the vertebra below.* For example, the spinous process of T8 is at the level of T9's transverse process.
4. <u>T10-T12</u> is as follows: [8 p.575]
   T10 follows the same rules as T7-T9.
   T11 follows the same rules as T4-T6.
   T12 follows the same rules as T1-T3.

B. Anatomical landmarks

The spine of the scapula corresponds with T3.
The inferior angle of the scapula corresponds with the spinous process of T7.
The sternal notch is level with T2. [1 p.530]

The sternal angle (angle of Louis) attaches to the 2nd rib is level with T4.[1 p.530]
The nipple is at the T4 dermatome.
The umbilicus is at the T10 dermatome.
The xiphisternal joint is anterior to T9. [1 p.530]

C. **Diaphrapm apertures** [1 p.536]

Vena cava at the level of T8
Esophageal hiatus at the level of T10
Aorta at the level of T12

II. **Thoracic motion**

A. The motions of the thoracic spine are rotation, sidebending, flexion and
extension. Motion is limited by the ribcage. *The main motion of the thorax is
rotation.* However, some authors suggest that lower segment (T11 and T12)
motion is similar to that of the lumbar region.

These authors report the following: [1 p.540]

Upper and middle thoracic: Rotation > flexion/extension> sidebending.

Lower thoracic: Flexion/extension > sidebending > rotation.

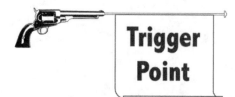

**Trigger
Point**

**Main motion of
the thoracic spine = Rotation.**

B. The thoracic spine follows Fryette's Laws (see Chapter 1 for details): [1 p.539]

If the spine is in the neutral position (no flexion or extension), and if
sidebending is introduced, rotation would then occur to the opposite side.
For example:
T5 - T10 Neutral, rotated right and sidebent left = T5 - T10 NR_RS_L

If the spine is in the non-neutral position (either flexed or extended), and
rotation is introduced, sidebending would then occur to the same side.
For example:
T5 Flexed, rotated right and sidebent right = T5 FR_RS_R

III. Muscles of Respiration

A. Primary muscles

1. Diaphragm

   Action:
      a. contracts with inspiration
      b. causes pressure gradients to help return lymph and venous blood back to the thorax

   Attachments: xyphoid process, ribs 6-12 on either side, and bodies and intervertebral discs of L1-L3

   Innervation: Phrenic nerve (C3-C5)

   Clinical importance: Somatic dysfunction of L1-L3 can be assocated with a flattened, ineffective, dysfunctional resting diaphragm. This alters pressure gradients and limits lymphatic return. [1 p.550]

2. Intercostals (external, internal, innermost, and subcostal)

   Action:
      a. elevate ribs during inspiration
      b. prevent retractions during inspiration

B. Secondary muscles

scalenes
pectoralis minor
serratus anterior and posterior
quadratus lumborum
latissimus dorsi

Ribcage

I. Anatomy

A. Typical vs. atypical ribs

What makes a typical rib typical?
A typical rib will have all of the following anatomical landmarks:

1. Tubercle – *articulates with the corresponding transverse process*
2. Head – *articulates with the vertebra above and corresponding vertebra*
3. Neck
4. Angle
5. Shaft

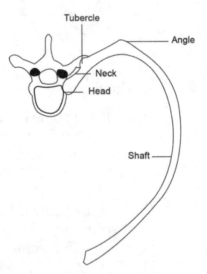

Fig 3.1: *Typical Rib*

A. Typical vs. atypical ribs (con't)

Typical ribs: 3-10
Atypical ribs: 1,2,11 and 12
NOTE: Sometimes rib 10 is
considered atypical. [3 p.37]

> Rib 1 – atypical because it
> articulates only with T1
> and has no angle
> Rib 2 – atypical because it has a
> large tuberosity on the
> shaft for the serratus
> anterior
> Rib 11 and 12 – atypical because
> they articulate
> only with the
> corresponding
> vertebrae and
> lack tubercles

> **MEMORY TOOL:**
> Atypical ribs have
> "1's" and "2's"
> Rib "1"
> Rib "2"
> Rib "11"
> Rib "12"
> Sometimes Rib "1"0

Rib 10 – sometimes considered atypical because it articulates only with T10

B. True, False and Floating Ribs

1. Ribs 1-7 - attach to the sternum through costal cartilages, therefore they are called **TRUE ribs**.
2. Ribs 8-12 – do not attach directly to the sternum, therefore they are called **FALSE ribs**. Each of the 8th to 10th ribs is connected by its costal cartilage to the cartilage of the rib superior. For example, the costal cartilage of rib 9 attaches to the costal cartiliage of rib 8. Ribs 11-12 remain unattached anteriorly and are often further classified as **FLOATING ribs**.

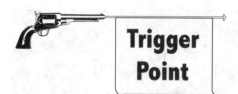

Trigger Point

> Know the difference
> between true, floating and
> false ribs.

II. Rib motion

There are three classifications of rib movement:

1. Pumphandle motion
2. Buckethandle motion
3. Caliper motion

NOTE: All ribs have a varying proportion of these motions depending on their location within the ribcage.

*The upper ribs (ribs 1-5) move **primarily** in a pump-handle motion.*
*The middle ribs (ribs 6-10) move **primarily** in a bucket-handle motion.*
*The lower ribs (ribs 11 and 12) move **primarily** in a caliper motion.*

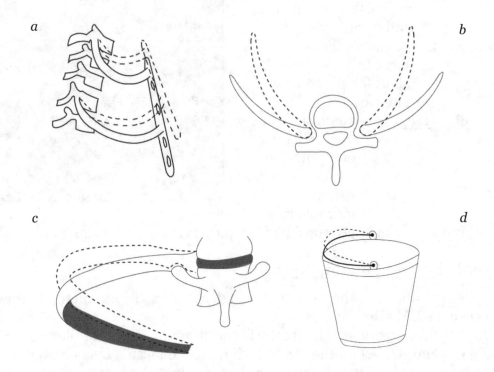

a

b

c

d

Fig 3.2a: *Pumphandle movement of ribs 1-5. The dotted lines show rib position in inhalation.*
Fig 3.2b: *Caliper motion of floating ribs. The dotted lines represent rib position in exhalation.*
Fig 3.2c: *Bucket-handle movement. A posterior-anterior view of a mid-thoracic rib. Note, that with inspiration, the rib moves up, similar to a bucket-handle.*

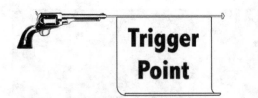

Trigger Point

Know the three different classifications of rib movement

III. <u>Rib Motion Testing</u> [1 p.422]

<u>Ribs 1 and 2 –</u>
Patient supine, physician palpates the sternoclavicular junction.
With the thumbs over the angle of rib 1, index finger posterior to the clavicle and middle or ring finger anterior to the clavicle.

Ribs 3-5
Patient supine, physician palpates the anterolateral aspect of the ribs.

Ribs 6-10
Patient supine, physician palpates the lateral aspects of the ribs (near mid axillary line).

Ribs 11-12
Patient prone, physician palpates ribs along rib shafts
Patient asked to inhale and exhale.

If the rib on the symptomatic side is statically cephalad and/or on inhalation has greater cephalad movement = **Inhalation dysfunction**
If the rib on the sympatomatic side is statically caudad and/or on exhalation has greater caudad movement = **Exhalation dysfunction**

IV. Rib dysfunctions:

Definition - A somatic dysfunction in which the movement or position of one rib is altered or disrupted. [1 p.1102]

The most common types of rib dysfunction are:
Inhalation Dysfunctions
Exhalation Dysfunctions

A. Inhalation dysfunction (older terminology: exhalation restriction)
The dysfunctional rib will move cephalad during inhalation; however the dysfunctional rib will not move caudad during exhalation.
The rib will therefore appear to be "held up."

Diagnostic Findings of Inhalation Dysfunction: [10 p.123, 129]

PUMP-HANDLE RIBS

Rib elevated: Anteriorly
Anterior part of rib moves cephalad on inspiration and is restricted on expiration.
Anterior narrowing of intercostal space above dysfunctional rib.
Superior edge of posterior rib angle is prominent.

Tenderness and Tissue Texture Changes
Costochondral junction
Chondrosternal junction
Posterior rib angles

BUCKET-HANDLE RIBS

Rib elevated: Laterally
Lateral part (shaft) of rib moves slightly upward on inspiration and is restricted on expiration.
Lateral narrowing of intercostal space above dysfunctional rib.
Lower edge of rib shaft is prominent.

Tenderness and Tissue Texture changes:
Intercostal muscles at mid-axillary line
Posterior rib angles

B. <u>Exhalation dysfunction</u> (older terminology: inhalation restriction)
The dysfunctional rib will move caudad during exhalation, however the dysfunctional rib will not move cephalad during inhalation.

Diagnostic Findings of Exhalation Dysfunction: [10 p.126, 131]

PUMP-HANDLE RIBS	BUCKET-HANDLE RIBS

<u>**Rib depressed:**</u> **Anteriorly**
  Anterior part of rib moves caudad on expiration and restricted on inspiration.
  Anterior narrowing of intercostal space below dysfunctional rib.
  Inferior edge of posterior rib angle is prominent.
 	
<u>Tenderness and Tissue Texture Changes</u>:
  Costochondral junction
  Chondrosternal junction
  Posterior rib angles
	<u>**Rib depressed:**</u> **Laterally**
	  Lateral part (shaft) of rib moves slightly downward on expiration and restricted on inspiration.
	  Lateral narrowing of intercostal space below dysfunctional rib.
	
	<u>Tenderness and Tissue Texture Changes</u>:
	  Intercostal muscles at mid-axillary line
	  Posterior rib angles

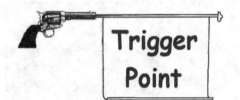

Trigger Point

> **Know the difference between inhalation and exhalation rib dysfunctions**

C. <u>Group dysfunctions</u>
<u>Definition</u> – An inhalation or exhalation rib dysfunction in which the movement or the position of two or more ribs is altered or disrupted.
    In these cases, there is usually one rib that is responsible for causing the dysfunction. This rib is referred to as the **"key"** rib.
*   In inhalation dysfunctions, the key rib is the lowest rib of the dysfunction. (see fig 3.3a)*
*   In exhalation dysfunctions, the key rib is the uppermost rib of the dysfunction. (see fig 3.3b)*

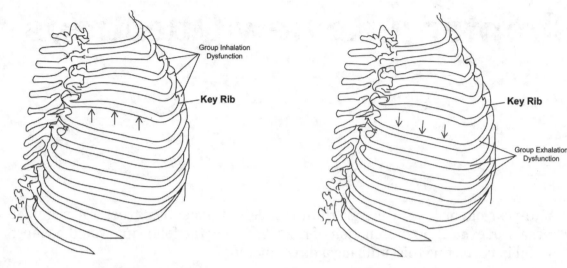

Fig 3.3a: *Group inhalation dysfunction*   **Fig 3.3b:** *Group exhalation dysfunction*

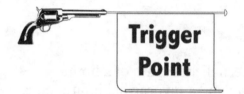

Know the "key" rib in group
and somatic dysfunction.

Treating a Group Dysfunction

   It is important to identify the key rib because, when treating a rib somatic dysfunction, treatment is directed towards the key rib. For example, if a patient has a group exhalation dysfunction of ribs 2 - 5, osteopathic treatment would be directed at rib 2.

MEMORY TOOL:

Key rib in group
dysfunctions:

BITE

B   bottom
I   inhalation
T   top
E   exhalation

Chapter 3 Review Questions

1. A 30-year-old male with allergic rhinitis sneezes frequently. Structural examination reveals an exhalation dysfunction of rib 2. Which of the following would be most useful in correcting this, utilizing a direct method?

   A. latissimus dorsi
   B. middle scalene
   C. pectoralis major
   D. pectoralis minor
   E. posterior scalene

2. A 54-year-old male presents with crushing, retrosternal chest pain of 2 hours' duration. He undergoes a comprehensive evaluation and a myocardial infarction is ruled out; however, some pain persists in the left chest. The discomfort is worse with extension, shoulder abduction, trunk movement, and there are tenderpoints in the pectoralis minor muscle. Dysfunction of which of the following could account for this clinical picture?

   A. rib 1
   B. rib 2
   C. ribs 3-5
   D. ribs 6-9
   E. rib 10

3. A 76-year-old male with an inoperable lung mass complains of rib pain and shortness of breath. He has been coughing up frothy, blood-tinged sputum during his frequent coughing bouts. Physical examination reveals coarse breath sounds. Ribs 5 and 6 on the right demonstrate reduced motion during inhalation. The most likely diagnosis is

   A. ribs 4-5 exhalation dysfunction
   B. ribs 5-6 exhalation dysfunction
   C. ribs 5-6 inhalation dysfunction
   D. ribs 6-7 exhalation dysfunction
   E. ribs 6-7 inhalation dysfunction

4. An 18-year-old female complains of a non-productive cough of 3 days' duration. She reports she was coughing so much that now her ribs are sore. Physical examination reveals she is febrile with scant rhonchi bilaterally. Structural examination reveals the right first rib is held in inhalation and ribs 7-10 on the left are held in exhalation. A likely cause of the right rib dysfunction is

    A. displacement by infiltrate
    B. intercostal muscle spasm
    C. pectoralis minor spasm
    D. scalene spasm
    E. somatovisceral reflex

Questions 5-9 are based on the following:
    A female with a history of asthma has been receiving osteopathic manipulative treatment to improve her costal cage motion.

5. In examining for bucket-handle motion of her ribs, the optimal placement of the operator's hands is over the

    A. angle of the ribs
    B. anterior margin of the ribs
    C. lateral border of the ribs
    D. sternum
    E. thoracic transverse processes

6. While assessing her physiologic motion of respiration, the operator palpates which primary muscle of respiration?

    A. external intercostals
    B. latissimus dorsi
    C. pectoralis minor
    D. quadratus lumborum
    E. scalenes

7. Which of the following are considered atypical ribs?

    A. 1, 2, 11, 12
    B. 1, 2, 9-12
    C. 1, 10-12
    D. 1-3, 11, 12
    E. 1-3, 10-12

8. The typical ribs are then palpated. Anatomic features consistent with a typical rib include

    A. articulation with the transverse process of the corresponding vertebra and the transverse process of the vertebra above
    B. costal groove for the azygos vein
    C. costosternal attachment
    D. one articular facet at the head of the rib
    E. one tubercle for articulation with the corresponding vertebral body

9. The operator lastly palpates the false ribs. The most appropriate list of ribs examined is

    A. 1-8
    B. 6-10
    C. 7-10
    D. 7-11
    E. 8-10

Questions 10-11 refer to the following:
   A 20-year-old female presents for a general maintenance examination without complaints. Structural examination reveals T10 is flexed, rotated and sidebent right.

10. The transverse process of this segment can be found

    A. at the level of the spinous process of T9
    B. at the level of the spinous process of T10
    C. at the level of the spinous process of T11
    D. halfway between the spinous processes of T9 and T10
    E. halfway between the spinous processes of T10 and T11

11. The associated dermatome at the level of T10 is at the

    A. anterior thigh just below the inguinal ligament
    B. epigastrium
    C. middle and anterior thigh
    D. suprapubic region
    E. umbilicus

Questions 12-13 refer to the following:
   A 40-year-old male reports right-sided thoracic pain after a work injury approximately one week ago. The pain has progressively improved; however, it is still present and exquisite at maximum inhalation. Structural examination reveals dysfunction of ribs 6-9. Radiographs are negative for fracture.

12. Which of the following statements describes the most appropriate diagnosis and treatment?

    A. exhalation dysfunction with treatment directed towards rib 6
    B. exhalation dysfunction with treatment directed towards rib 9
    C. inhalation dysfunction with treatment directed towards rib 6
    D. inhalation dysfunction with treatment directed towards rib 9
    E. torsional dysfunction with treatment directed towards rib 9

13. The physician elects to perform muscle energy to the treatment area. The most appropriate muscle to activate is the

    A. latissimus dorsi
    B. pectoralis major
    C. pectoralis minor
    D. quadratus lumborum
    E. serratus anterior

Questions 14-15 refer to the following:

A 35-year-old male presents with chest pain after a horse kicked him in the right anterior chest wall. The pain is worse with inhalation. Physical examination reveals the lungs are clear to auscultation and ribs without point tenderness. Structural examination reveals the following:

- Increased intercostal space between ribs 2 and 3 anteriorly on the right
- Inferior edge of rib angle prominent from ribs 3-7
- Decreased excursion of ribs 3-7 on the right during inhalation

Plain film radiography is negative for fracture.

14. The most likely dysfunction in ribs 3-7 on the right is

    A. exhalation somatic dysfunction, bucket-handle predominant
    B. exhalation somatic dysfunction, pump-handle predominant
    C. inhalation somatic dysfunction, bucket-handle predominant
    D. inhalation somatic dysfunction, pump-handle predominant
    E. torsional somatic dysfunction, bucket-handle predominant

15. Which of the following muscles will most likely assist in treating these ribs with muscle energy treatment?

    A. anterior scalene
    B. serratus posterior
    C. pectoralis minor
    D. posterior scalenes
    E. serratus anterior

Explanations

1. Answer: **E**

   An exhalation dysfunction has a restriction in inhalation. The posterior scalene muscle attaches to ribs 2 and would be best used to augment treatment. The anterior and middle scalene are used to treat to rib 1, the pectoralis minor is used to treat ribs 3-5, the serratus anterior is used to treat ribs 6-9, latissimus dorsi is used to treat ribs 10-11, and quadratus lumborum is used to treat rib 12. Refer to Chapter 15 Muscle Energy for more information about treatment.

2. Answer: **C**

   It is always important to rule out obvious, non-cardiac causes of chest pain such as costochondritis or somatic dysfunction. Since this patient has exquisite tenderness in the pectoralis minor muscle, which attaches to ribs 3-5, it is possible that an associated rib 3-5 dysfunction is contributory.

3. Answer: **B**

   Somatic dysfunction is named for the freedom of motion. Since this patient's ribs move freely into exhalation it is called an exhalation dysfunction.

4. Answer: **D**

   The anterior and middle scalenes attach to rib 1 and if strained from coughing may contribute to rib dysfunction of its associated attachment. Ribs are unlikely to be displaced by infiltrates. The first intercostal muscle is located between ribs 1 and 2, and spasm will not cause a inhalation dysfunction of rib 1. A somatovisceral reflex occurs when a somatic dysfunction contributes to segmentally-related visceral dysfunction (e.g., rib dysfunction causing a pulmonary issue).

5. Answer: **C**

   The most appropriate means to assess bucket handle motion of ribs 6-10 while facing the patient is to place your hands over the lateral borders of the rib cage with fingers pointing posteriorly and aligned with the patient's intercostal spaces. Ribs 1 and 2 are assessed with the physician palpating the sternoclavicular junction. Ribs 3-5 are evaluated with the physician palpating the mid-clavicular line. Ribs 11 and 12 are evaluated with the patient prone while palpating along the shafts of the ribs.

6. Answer: **A**

Primary muscles of respiration include the diaphragm and intercostals: internal, external, and subcostal. All of the other options are secondary muscles of respiration.

7. Answer: **A**

Atypical ribs have features that are not consistent with the majority of ribs. Rib 1 only articulates with the body of T1. Rib 2 has a large tuberosity and only one synovial joint attaching to the body of the sternum. Some consider rib 10 to be atypical since it only articulates with T10 and not T9. Ribs 11 and 12 do not articulate with the costosternal cartilage at all.

8. Answer: **C**

Typical ribs have two articular facets on the head of the rib that articulates with the corresponding vertebral body as well as the one above. The tubercle articulates with the corresponding transverse process only (not the transverse process of the above vertebra). The azygous vein is a large vessel on the right side in the posterior thorax that drains into the superior vena cava. Note that ribs 11 and 12 do not have anterior attachments and do not articulate with the transverse process of the vertebra of their corresponding level. All typical ribs have costosternal attachments (including some atypical ribs).

9. Answer: **E**

True ribs attach to the sternum and consist of ribs 1-7. All other ribs below this level are either connected through costal cartilage or are floating (ribs 11 and 12).

10. Answer: **A**

This question uses the 'Rule of Three's' in reverse and is essentially asking which spinous process can be found at the level of T10. Finding the spinous process of T10 follows the same rules as T7-T9 in which the spinous processes are located at the level of the transverse process of the vertebra below. Therefore, the spinous process of T9 will be present at the level of the T10 transverse processes.

11. Answer: **E**

The T10 dermatome is at the level of the umbilicus. T11 is below the umbilicus while T12 is just above the inguinal ligament in the suprapubic region. The L1 nerve root has sensation in the anterior thigh below the inguinal ligament, while the L2 root innervates the middle and anterior thigh.

12. Answer: **A**

The dysfunction is considered an exhalation dysfunction if it has freer motion with exhalation and is restricted with inhalation. Treatment should focus on the key rib of this group, rib 6, since it is an exhalation dysfunction. This can be remembered by the mnemonic BITE for 'Bottom Inhaled, Top Exhaled.'

13. Answer: **E**

The serratus anterior would be best utilized to augment treatment on rib 6 (key rib). The anterior and middle scalene are used to treat to rib 1, the pectoralis minor is used to treat ribs 3-5, the serratus anterior is used to treat ribs 6-9, the latissimus dorsi is used to treat ribs 10-11, and the quadratus lumborum is used to treat rib 12. Refer to Chapter 15 Muscle Energy for more information about treatment.

14. Answer: **B**

The patient has an exhalation dysfunction due to freer motion during exhalation with restriction during inhalation. Ribs 1-5 primarily move in a pump-handle motion while ribs 6-10 primarily move in a bucket-handle motion. The majority of the ribs in question have a predominantly pump handle motion. The question stem cites that the intercostal space between ribs 2-3 is increased because ribs 3-7 have move in exhalation when inferior compared to ribs 1-2. In a pump handle dysfunction the inferior edge of the corresponding rib angles will be prominent.

15. Answer: **C**

The pectoralis minor attaches to ribs 3-5 and would be used to treat the key rib (in this case, rib 3). The anterior and middle scalene are used to treat to rib 1, the pectoralis minor is used to treat ribs 3-5, the serratus anterior is used to treat ribs 6-9, the latissimus dorsi is used to treat ribs 10-11, and the quadratus lumborum is used to treat rib 12. Refer to Chapter 15 Muscle Energy for more information about treatment.

LUMBAR SPINE 4

I. Anatomy

A. Important clinical points

There are five lumbar vertebrae distinguishable by their large quadrangular spinous processes. The large cross-sectional area of the lumbar vertebral body is designed to sustain longitudinal loads.[8 p.582]

The posterior longitudinal ligament runs vertically along the posterior aspect of the vertebral body. *This ligament begins to narrow at the lumbar region.* At L4 and L5 the posterior longitudinal ligament is one-half the width of that at L1. This narrowing produces a weakness in the posteriolateral aspect of the intervertebral disc. *This weakness makes the lumbar spine more susceptible to disc herniations.*

The iliolumbar ligament originates from the transverse processes of L4 and L5 and inserts onto the iliac crest and superior portion of the SI joint. *This ligament is typically the first ligament to become tender with lumbosacral stress or decompensation.*[1 p.550]

In the thoracic and lumbar region *a nerve root will exit the intervertebral foramen below its corresponding vertebra (see fig 4.1).*

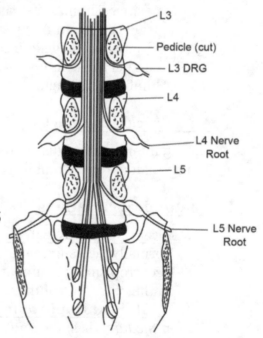

Fig 4.1: *(DRG = Dorsal Root Ganglion) Lumbar nerve roots exit intervertebral foramen below the corresponding vertebrae, but above the intervertebral disc.*

For example, the L4 nerve root will exit the spinal column between L4 and L5. The spinal cord usually terminates between L1 and L2. Therefore, the exiting nerve roots become longer as they approach the lower segments, causing *the lumbar nerve roots to exit the superior aspect of their corresponding intervertebral foramina, just **above** the intervertebral disc.* This information is important when considering disc herniations (discussed later).

B. **Muscles**

Erector spinae group (spinalis, longissimus, iliocostalis)

Multifidus and rotatores

Quadratus lumborum

Iliopsoas – composed of the psoas major muscle and iliacus muscle.

> **Origin** – T12 - L5 vertebral bodies[5] p.385
>
> **Insertion** – Lesser trochanter of femur
>
> **Action** – primary flexor of the hip
>
> **Clinical importance** – Somatic dysfunction of the iliopsoas muscle is very common, and is usually precipitated from prolonged shortening of the muscle. A pelvic side shift, positive Thomas test, and somatic dysfunction of an upper lumbar segment is commonly seen with iliopsoas dysfunctions (for further discussion see flexion contracture of the iliopsoas - Section IV C in this chapter). The iliopsoas also plays an important role in maintaining the lumbosacral angle.

> **MEMORY TOOL:**[13 p.3 4]
>
> Erector spinae group = "SILO"
> S = Spinalis
> I = Iliocostalis
> LO = LOngissimus

C. **Anatomical landmarks**

L4 - L5 intervertebral disc at the level of the iliac crest.
T10 dermatome at the umbilicus, which is anterior to L3 and L4 intervertebral disc.

D. **Anatomical variations**

1. Facet (zygopophyseal) Trophism – An asymmetry of the facet joint angles. Normally facets in the lumbar spine are aligned in the sagittal plane. In facet tropism, one lumbar facet will not match the orientation of the facet on the other side of the corresponding vertebra.
   Clinical Importance – This is considered the *most common anomaly in the lumbar spine and is found in 30% of patients.*[7 p.449, 1 p.548] This may also predispose to early degenerative changes. [11]

2. <u>Sacralization</u> – a bony deformity in which one or both of the transverse processes of L5 are long and articulate with the sacrum. Sacralization is present in 3.5% of individuals,[12 p.367] and may alter the structure-function relationship of the lumbosacral junction, leading to early disc degeneration.

3. <u>Lumbarization</u> – most often occurs from the failure of fusion of S1 with the other sacral segments. Lumbarization is much less common than sacralization.

4. <u>Spina Bifida</u> – a developmental anomaly in which there is a defect in the closure of the lamina of the vertebral segment. It usually occurs in the lumbar spine. There are three types of spina bifida:

   a. **<u>Spina bifida occulta</u>** – No herniation through the defect. Often the only physical sign of this anomaly is a course patch of hair over the site.
   b. **<u>Spina bifida meningocele</u>** – A herniation of the meninges through the defect.
   c. **<u>Spina bifida meningomyelocele</u>** – A herniation of the meninges and the nerve roots through the defect; associated with neruological deficits.

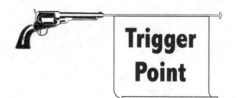

Know the definition and different types of Spina Bifida.

II. <u>Lumbar mechanics and somatic dysfunction</u>

Due to the alignment of the facets (backward and medial for the superior facets), *the major motion of the lumbar spine is flexion and extension.* There is a small degree of sidebending and a very limited amount of rotation. Motion of the lumbar spine will follow Fryette's laws. Somatic dysfunction may occur in any of the three planes of motion. It is not uncommon to find that a single segment dysfunction does not follow Fryette's principles, especially L5.[1.p.564]

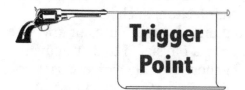

Main motion of the lumbar spine = Flexion/Extension

A. In sacral torsions, motion of L5 will influence the motion of the sacrum in two ways:[1 p.590]

1. Sidebending of L5 will cause a sacral oblique axis to be engaged on the same side.

2. Rotation of the L5 will cause the sacrum to rotate toward the opposite side.

For a further description of the influence of L5 on lumbosacral mechanics, see Chapter 6 Sacrum and Innominates.

III. <u>Lumbosacral angle (Ferguson's angle)</u> (see fig 4.3)

The lumbosacral angle is formed by the intersection of a horizontal line and the line of inclination of the sacrum. This angle is normally between 25° and 35°. [14 p.164] An increase in Ferguson's angle causes a shear stress placed on the lumbosacral joint, often causing low back pain.

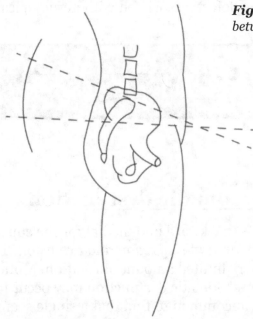

Fig 4.3: Ferguson's angle: The angle formed between the two dotted lines (normally 25° -35°).

IV. <u>Causes of low back pain</u>

Low back pain may be acute or chronic. Acute causes of low back pain may be due to fracture, recent strain or disc herniation, an infection, such as osteomyelitis or meningitis, or it may be referred pain. Chronic causes of low back pain are much more common. It is important as a physician to distinguish between congenital, metabolic, neoplastic, and degenerative cause of low back pain. Since there are several causes of low back pain, our discussion will be limited to the mechanical causes of low back pain. Although not very common, another important cause of low back pain is cauda equina syndrome, which will also be discussed.

A. <u>Somatic dysfunctions of the lumbosacral spine (back strain/sprain)</u>

<u>Location of back pain</u>: low back, buttock, posterior lateral thigh [15 p.183]

<u>Quality of pain</u>: ache, muscle spasm [15 p.183]

<u>Signs and symptoms</u>: increased pain with activity or prolonged standing or sitting, increased muscle tension

<u>Treatment</u>: OMT consisting of counterstrain for tenderpoints, muscle energy or HVLA for restrictions. OMT should also be directed at decreasing restrictions in other areas that may alter the structure-function relationship of the lumbosacral spine.

B. <u>Psoas syndrome (a.k.a. flexion contracture of the iliopsoas)</u>[3 p.747]

<u>Pathogenesis</u>: often precipitated from prolonged positions that shorten the psoas.[3 p.747] However, organic causes may also cause psoas spasm through viscero-somatic or somato-somatic reflexes. Organic causes must be ruled out before initiating treatment for mechanical causes.

<u>Organic causes include</u>:[3 p.747, 7 p.484, 1 p.572]
1. Appendicitis
2. Sigmoid colon dysfunction
3. Ureteral calculi
4. Endometriosis
5. Ureter dysfunction
6. Metastatic carcinoma of the prostate
7. Salpingitis

<u>Location of pain</u>: low back sometimes radiating to groin

<u>Quality of pain</u>: ache, muscle spasm

<u>Signs and symptoms</u>: restricted hip extension, increased pain when standing or walking, positive Thomas test, tender point 1 cm medial to ASIS, [1 p.594] *nonneutral dysfunction of L1 or L2, positive pelvic shift test to the contralateral side, lumbar hyperlordosis, and contralateral piriformis spasm.* [1 p.623]

<u>Treatment</u>:[8 p.489] An acute spasm may benefit from ice to decrease pain and edema. Do not initially use heat. Counterstrain to the anterior iliopsoas tenderpoint is very effective followed by muscle energy or HVLA to the high lumbar dysfunction. *Some authors[7] report that symptoms will not resolve until the high lumbar dysfunction is treated.*

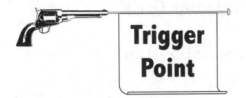

Trigger Point

> A flexion contracture of the iliopsoas is often associated with a nonneutral dysfunction of L1 or L2.

C. Iliolumbar Ligament syndrome[1 p.573]

<u>Pathogenesis</u>: Iliolumbar ligament becomes stressed, irritated and painful. Occurs with acute L5 disc protrusion, spinal instability, or spondylolisthiesis.

<u>Signs and symptoms</u>: Tissue texture change at the ilial insertion of the ligament. Pelvic sideshift toward the iliolumbar lilgaments. Ipsilateral adductor muscle tight.

<u>Treatment</u>: Counterstrain to iliolumbar ligament has significant clinical value.

D. Herniated nucleus pulposus

<u>Pathogenesis</u>: Due to the narrowing of the posterior longitudinal ligament, a posteriolateral herniation of the intervertebral disc is a common problem. 98% of herniations occur between L4 and L5, or between L5 and S1.[15 p.191] *A posteriolateral herniated disc in the lumbar region will typically exert pressure on the nerve root of the vertebrae below.*

For example, a posterio-latareal herniation between L3 and L4 will affect the nerve root of L4 (see fig 4.4).

<u>Location of pain</u>: lower back and lower leg

<u>Quality of pain</u>: Numbness and/or tingling which may be accompanied by sharp, burning and/or shooting pain radiating down the leg, and typically worsens with flexion of the lumbar spine.

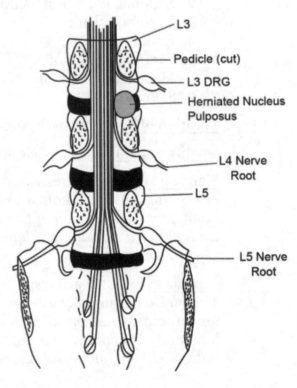

Fig 4.4: Herniated Nucleus Pulposus. Herniated disc at L3/L4 will likely exert pressure on L4 nerve root.

53

<u>Signs and Symptoms</u>: weakness and decreased reflexes associated with the affected nerve root. Sensory deficit over the corresponding dermatome. Positive straight leg raising test.

<u>Radiology</u>: MRI is the gold standard.

<u>Treatment</u>: Most cases can be treated conservatively. Bed rest for no more than 2 days.[16] OMT - Initially indirect techniques, followed by gentle direct. *HVLA is relatively contraindicated.* Physical therapy, pharmacotherapy (NSAIDS, muscle relaxers, neuropathic agents, opiates). Epidural sterorid injections Surgical decompression is considered if conservative treatment fails.

E. **Spinal stenosis**

<u>Definition</u>: Narrowing of the spinal canal or intervertebral foramina usually due to degenerative changes, causing pressure on nerve roots (or rarely the cord).[17 p.540]

<u>Pathogenesis</u>: Degenerative changes in the lumbar spine can include:
1) Hypertrophy of the facet joints or ligamentum flavum.
2) Broad based disc bulge, protrusion or herniation.
3) Loss of intervertebral disc height.

All of which can narrow the spinal canal and/or intervertebral foramina and result in nerve root compression.

<u>Location of pain</u>: Lower back to legs.

<u>Quality of pain</u>: ache, shooting pain or paresthesias.

<u>Signs and symptoms</u>: Worsened by lumbar extension (standing, walking or lying supine).

<u>Radiology</u>: osteophytes and decreased intervertebral disc space are usually present. MRI demonstrating central or foraminal stenosis.

<u>Treatment</u>: OMT should be directed at decreasing any restrictions, improving range of motion and releasing any lumbar extensor spasm. Additional conservative management includes physical therapy, NSAID's or low dose tapering steroids. An epidural steroid injection may be used if conservative therapy is not effective. Surgical laminectomy with decompression is indicated if above fails.

F. <u>Spondylosis</u> (see fig 4.5) –
A radiographical term for
degenerative changes within the
intervertebral disc and ankylosing of
adjacent vertebral bodies.[8 p.1138]

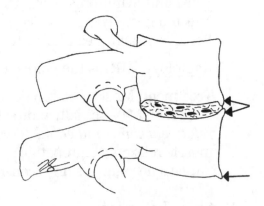

Fig 4.5: *Spondylosis: Three arrows show the anterior lipping of the vertebral bodies. Note the associated degenerative changes within the intervertebral disc.*

G. <u>Spondylolysis</u> (see fig 4.6) – a
defect usually of the pars
interarticularis **without** anterior
displacement of the vertebral
body. Symptoms and treatment
are similar to spondylolisthesis.
Since lateral lumbar x-rays will
not reveal any slippage, **oblique
views will identify the
fracture of the pars
interarticularis. It is often
seen as a "collar" on the neck
of the scotty dog**.

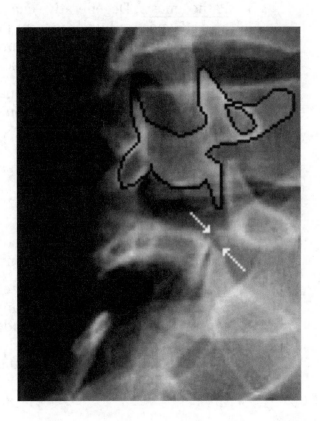

Fig 4.6: *Oblique view of the lumbar spine. Black outline demonstrates the scotty dog. White arrows show lucency (a black collar around the neck of the scootty dog) in the pars interarticularis in the vertebra below.*

H. <u>Spondylolisthesis</u> (see fig 4.7)

<u>Definition</u>: *anterior displacement* of one vertebra in relation to the one below.[8 p.1138] Often occurs at L4 or L5. This can an be due to bilateral fractures in the pars (usually at L5/S1), or can be related to degeneration of the facet joints from longstanding instability (usually at L4/5).[1 p.475]

<u>Prevalence</u>: 5% of the population. However, approximately half are asymptomatic. Patients who become symptomatic do so usually after the age of 20.[7vp.366]

<u>Location of pain</u>: low back, buttock and/or posterior thigh.[6 p.368]

<u>Quality of pain</u>: ache.

<u>Signs and symptoms</u>: Increased pain with extension-based activities. Tight hamstrings bilaterally. Stiffed-legged, short-stride, waddling type gait. [8 p.1009, 7 p.367, 1 p.476] Typically, there are no neurologic deficits. *Positive vertebral step-off sign (palpating the spinous processes there is an obvious anterior displacement at the area of the listhesis).*

<u>Radiology</u>: anterior displacement of one vertebrae on another seen on lateral films. Can be classified (grade 1 - 4) based on the degree of slippage (see figure 4.5)

<u>Treatment</u>: most patients (85 - 90%) can be managed with conservative management. The goals of manipulation is to reduce lumbar lordosis and somatic dysfunction [1 p.479] *HVLA is relatively contraindicated.*[1 p.479] Additional conservative management includes weight loss, avoiding high heels and avoiding flexion based exercises.[7 p.371-74] Heel lifts have been advocated to control postural mechanics. Lumbo-sacral orthotics can be considered for short term stability.[8 p.1012]

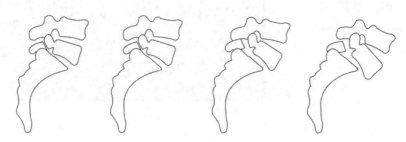

GRADE I   GRADE II   GRADE III   GRADE IV

Fig 4.7:   *Grading of Spondylolisthesis.*
Grade 1 = 0 - 25%
Grade 2 = 25 - 50%
Grade 3 = 50 - 75%
Grade 4 = >75%

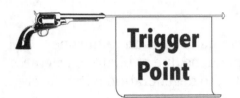

Trigger Point

Know the difference between spondylolisthesis, spondylolysis, and spondylosis

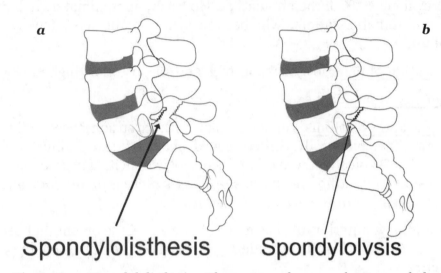

a   *b*

Spondylolisthesis   Spondylolysis

Fig 4.8a: *Spondylolisthesis   The arrow shows a fracture of the pars interarticularis with anterior displacement of L5 on the sacrum.*
Fig 4.8b: *Spondylolysis   The arrow shows a fracture of the pars interarticularis without anterior displacement.*

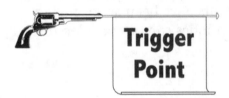

Trigger Point

Diagnose:

1) Spondylolisthesis with lateral x-rays

2) Spondylolysis with oblique x-rays

I. Cauda Equina Syndrome[15 p.682, 18 p.481, 1 p.566]

<u>Definition</u>: pressure on the nerve roots of the cauda equina usually due to a massive central disc herniation, spondylolisthesis, fracture or tumor

<u>Location of pain</u>: low back and legs

<u>Quality of pain</u>: sharp

<u>Radiology</u>: MRI is the gold standard

<u>Signs and symptoms</u>: Saddle anesthesia, decreased deep tendon reflexes, decreased rectal sphincter tone, and loss of bowel and bladder control

<u>Treatment</u>: Emergent surgical decompression of the cauda equina is imperative (within 48 hours). If surgery is delayed too long, permanent neurologic damage can ensue

Chapter 4 Review Questions

1. A young male presents for a routine physical. His structural examination is unremarkable. You evaluate the patient's lumbar range of motion and note the main motion to be

   A. flexion and extension
   B. rotation
   C. sidebending
   D. sidebending and rotation
   E. translation

2. A newborn is delivered with a posterior lumbar mass. Ultrasound revealed that the mass appears to be composed of meningeal and neural tissue. The most likely diagnosis is

   A. disc herniation
   B. spina bifida meningocele
   C. spina bifida meningomyelocele
   D. spina bifida occulta
   E. spondylolysis

3. A 55-year-old male presents to your office with low back pain radiating to his lower extremities. He states that yesterday his feet felt numb and weak, and now this feeling has progressed into his thighs. Neuromuscular examination reveals 0+ deep tendon reflexes in the lower extremities bilaterally, 3/5 muscle strength in the ankle plantar flexors, 3/5 in ankle dorsiflexors, and 3/5 in knee flexors and extensors. Digital rectal examination reveals decreased rectal tone. The most likely cause is

   A. a spinal cord mass effect above the level of L1
   B. compression of the thecal sac
   C. epidural venous plexus congestion
   D. meningeal inflammation
   E. severe spondylolysis

4. A 70-year-old male presents with chronic radicular low back pain associated with bilateral lower extremity pain and paresthesia. Which of the following additional findings is most closely associated with this clinical presentation?

    A. increased pain with standing and walking
    B. extensor plantar response
    C. fasciculations
    D. increased deep tendon reflexes
    E. symmetrical proximal hip girdle

5. A 25-year-old male complains of low back pain. History reveals it is worse with forward bending. Structural examination reveals the right transverse process of L2 becomes more posterior with flexion. The most appropriate nomenclature for this dysfunction is

    A. ER_LS_L
    B. ER_RS_R
    C. FR_LS_L
    D. FR_RS_R
    E. NR_RS_L

6. A young male presents with back pain. Observation reveals he is standing in a flexed, sidebent right posture. Physical examination findings include resisted hip extension on the right, a tenderpoint medial to the right ASIS. The most likely cause is

    A. piriformis tension on the side of the discomfort
    B. S1 nerve root compression
    C. sciatic nerve compression under the inguinal ligament
    D. spondylolysis of the L3-L4 segments
    E. hypertonic right psoas muscle

7. A 55-year-old plumber presents with chronic low back pain. Structural examination in the prone position reveals the following:

- Boggy area over the paravertebral tissue at L1 right
- Resistance to anterior motion over the right transverse process of L1
- Resistance to anterior motion over the spinous process of L1

The most likely diagnosis is

    A. L1 ERS_L
    B. L1 ERS_R
    C. L1 FRS_L
    D. L1 FRS_R
    E. L1 NR_LS_R

<u>The following information pertains to questions 8-9</u>:

A 65-year-old machinist presents with chronic low back pain. History reveals he must spend several hours in a forward bent position while working. Structural examination reveals a hypertonic left psoas.

8. The most likely associated postural screening finding is

    A. elevated right iliac crest
    B. flexed L5 dysfunction
    C. sacral shear
    D. pelvic side shift right
    E. posterior left sacrum

9. The most likely associated somatic dysfunction is

    A. L1 FRS$_L$
    B. L2 ERS$_R$
    C. L3 FRS$_R$
    D. L5 FRS$_L$
    E. posterior sacrum left

<u>The following information pertain to questions 10 -12</u> :

For each numbered item (objective finding) select one heading (diagnosis) most closely associated with it. Each lettered heading may be selected once, more than once, or not at all.

    A. spina bifida
    B. spinal stenosis
    C. spondylolisthesis
    D. spondylolysis
    E. spondylosis

10. The anterior displacement of one vertebral body in relation to the one below is known as

    A. A
    B. B
    C. C
    D. D
    E. E

11. Degenerative changes within the intervertebral disc and ankylosing of adjacent vertebral bodies is known as

    A. A
    B. B
    C. C
    D. D
    E. E

12. A lumbar spine roentgenogram reveals a 'collar around the neck of the Scotty dog' at L5.

    A. A
    B. B
    C. C
    D. D
    E. E

The following information pertain to questions 13-15:
    For each numbered item (objective finding) select one heading (affected nerve root) most closely associated with it. Each lettered heading may be selected once, more than once, or not at all.

    A. L2
    B. L3
    C. L4
    D. L5
    E. S1

13. An MRI of the lumbar spine reveals severe stenosis of the intervertebral foramen affecting the nerve root between L3 and L4.

    A. A
    B. B
    C. C
    D. D
    E. E

14. Physical examination reveals an absent patellar reflex with associated sensory loss down the medial aspect of the leg.

    A. A
    B. B
    C. C
    D. D
    E. E

15. An MRI of the lumbar spine reveals a posteriolateral disc herniation of the intervertebral disc of L4-L5.

    A. A
    B. B
    C. C
    D. D
    E. E

Explanations

1. Answer: **A**

    The major motion of the lumbar spine is flexion and extension due to the orientation of the facets in the sagittal plane. There is a small degree of sidebending and a limited amount of rotation in the lumbar spine.

2. Answer: **C**

    In spina bifida meningomyelocele the lamina defect is usually large and allows the spinal cord (myelo-) to protrude through the defect as opposed to the meninges alone. This form of spina bifida is often associated with neurologic defects. A disc herniation will not result in a posterior lumbar mass. Spondylolysis is caused by a defect in the pars interarticularis. In spina bifida occulta, the only physical sign is a course patch of hair over the site. In spina bifida meningocele, there is a herniation through the lamina defect; however the sac would not contain any neural elements.

3. Answer: **B**

    Cauda equina syndrome, also known as epidural spinal cord compression or ESCC, is due to compression of the thecal sac of the spinal cord. It is commonly caused by a growing malignant neoplasm but may also be caused by lumbar spinal stenosis from a vertebral body due to a spondylolisthesis, a compression fracture or a severe disc herniation. In adults, the tip of the spinal cord (conus medullaris) usually lies at the L1 vertebral level. The cauda equina is the bundle of nerves and spinal roots below this level, and compression of these structures results in the symptoms mentioned in the stem and explanation below. Note that hyperreflexia is typically more common with lesions above the cauda equina, which is the main reason that distractor A is incorrect. Epidural venous plexus congestion can be due to inferior vena cava occlusion, this has not been associated with decreased rectal tone. Meningeal inflammation and severe spondyolysis will not present with the above neurological deficits.

4. Answer: **A**

    In patients with spinal stenosis, symptoms are often worsened with standing and walking. Standing and walking narrows the spinal canal and neural foramen. Therefore any structure causing stenosis can result in neural compression with standing and walking. Extensor plantar response (Babinski's sign), fasiculations, and increased deep tendon reflexes are seen in upper motor neuron lesions. Although weakness in the hip girdle could arise from an upper lumbar stenosis, stenosis in the lower lumbar segments is much more common.

5. Answer: **B**

    In this patient, the right transverse process of L2 becomes more posterior with flexion. Therefore, L2 is likely extended and rotated right. Since the asymmetry worsens with flexion, Fryette's type II mechanics apply, and L2 must sidebend in the same direction of rotation.

6. Answer: **E**

    Psoas syndrome is associated with ipsilateral restricted hip extension, increased pain when standing or walking, (often the patient will stand flexed and sidebent to the side of the shortened psoas) positive Thomas test, tender point 1 cm medial to ASIS, nonneutral dysfunction of L1 or L2, positive pelvic shift test to the contralateral side, sacral dysfunction on an oblique axis, and contralateral piriformis spasm.

7. Answer: **D**

    Somatic dysfunction is named for the freedom of motion. This patient's L1 is flexed because it is noted to have resistance with anterior motion over the spinous process which induced extension. The L1 is rotated right because it has resistance with left rotation as noted when applying anterior pressure to the right transverse process. Since it is flexed and rotated right, it must be sidebent right.

8. Answer: **D**

    Psoas syndrome is due to a psoas spasm that can cause a persistent strain across the lumbosacral junction and is associated with a constellation of signs and symptoms. The pelvic side shift test, like all somatic dysfunctions, is named positive to the side of freer motion. In a contracted psoas on the left, the pelvis will shift to the right, resulting in a positive pelvic shift test to the right. Psoas syndrome is also associated with an L1 or L2 somatic dysfunction (not necessarily L5). Although some authors reported a sacral dysfunction on an oblique axis associated with psoas syndrome, [3 p.747] sacral shear and posterior sacrum have not been reported. Other signs include flexed posture sidebent to the affected side, a positive Thomas test, enhanced lumbar lordosis, and tenderpoints of the ipsilateral iliacus and contralateral piriformis. [1 p.623]

9. Answer: **A**

    The L1 or L2 vertebra is commonly flexed and rotated to the affected side.

10. Answer: **C**

    Spondylolisthesis involves anterior displacement of a vertebral body. This can be due to bilateral defects of the posterior arch (pars interarticularis) or related to degeneration of the facet joints.

11. Answer: **E**

Spondylosis is a general term for nonspecific, degenerative changes of the spine.

12. Answer: **D**

Spondylolysis is a unilateral or bilateral defect (fracture or separation) in the vertebral pars interarticularis, without anterior displacement of the vertebrae. It is most common in athletes who engage in sports involving extreme spinal motion, particularly lumbar extension. A roentgenogram is another name for an x-ray.

13. Answer: **B**

Nerve roots exit at the level below their associated vertebra starting at T1 (note that C8 is between C7 and T1) through the intervertebral foramen. Compression of structures within the intervertebral foramen will compress the L3 nerve root between the L3 and L4 vertebrae.

14. Answer: **C**

The L4 nerve root can be tested by assessing the patellar deep tendon reflex, ankle dorsiflexion, and sensation along the medial leg and malleolus. Refer to Appendix B to review dermatomes and motor functions of the lumbar spine.

15. Answer: **D**

This is a challenging concept. Depending upon the nature and location of intraspinal compression (central, posteriolateral or lateral), nerve roots may be injured at any disc level, from the L1-2 level where the spinal cord ends as the conus medullaris to the level of their exit into their neural foramina. The L5 root can be compressed by a central disc protrusion at L2-3 or L3-4, a posteriolateral disc protrusion at the L4-5 level, or a lateral disc protrusion into the foramen at L5-S1.

SCOLIOSIS AND SHORT LEG SYNDROME 5

Scoliosis

I. Definition

1) an appreciable lateral deviation of the spine from the normally straight vertical line of the spine.[19] 2) a pathological or functional lateral curve of the spine.[1 p.1106] Due to Fryette's laws, any sidebending of the spine will automatically induce rotation. Therefore, the term "rotoscoliosis" is thought to be more accurate.

A. Epidemiology – 5% of school-age children develop scoliosis by age 15.[7 p.350] however, only 10% of those children have clinical symptoms related to their scoliotic curvatures.[7 p.350]
Female: Male ratio = 4:1.

B. Naming scoliosis –

Curve that is sidebent left = scoliosis to the right (convexity on the right)= dextroscoliosis. (see fig 4.1a)
Dextro - donoting a relationship to the right.[19]

Curve that is sidebent right = scoliosis to the left (convexity on the left) = levoscoliosis. (see fig 4.1b)
Levo - donoting a relationship to the left.[19]

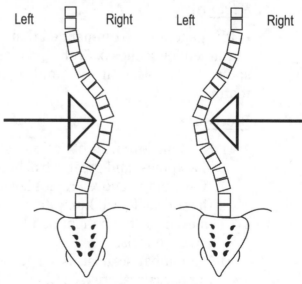

Fig 5.1a: *Dextroscoliosis* ***Fig 5.1b:*** *Levoscoliosis*

67

> ## MEMORY TOOL:
>
> The arrow in figure 5.1a points to the right in Dextroscoliosis
>
> The arrow in figure 5.1b points to the left in Levoscoliosis

II.
Classification of scoliosis curves

Two Types

1) Structural Curve:[1 p.467, 21 p.433]

   A spinal curve that is relatively fixed and inflexible. a structural curve will not correct with sidebending in the opposite direction. it is associated with vertebral wedging and shortened ligaments and muscles on the concave side of the curve. Structural curves will not reduce with lift therapy.[61 p.443]

2) Functional Curve:[1 p.467, 21 p.433]

   A spinal curve that is flexible and can be partially or completely corrected with sidebending to the opposite side. an uncorrected functional curve may eventually progress into a structural curve.

III. Screening and measuring scoliosis [1 p.451,456,467]

A. Screening

It is generally recommended that children ages 10 - 15 years old be examined for scoliosis. Scoliosis often increases rapidly during the growth spurt of an adolescent[1 p.467-8] and stabilizes when the patient reaches skeletal maturity.

Procedure

1) Examine levelness of occiput, shoulders, iliac crests, posterior superior iliac spines, and greater trochanters.
2) If any of the above are not level, have the patient bend forward at the waist. If a rib hump (a group of ribs that appear higher on one side as the patient bends forward) appears, the patient is likely to have scoliosis.
3) If a lumbar scoliosis is suspected, utilize the hip drop test to evaluate for lumbar curvature (see Chapter 18 Special Tests)

B. Measuring scoliotic curves

Spinal curves are measured with x-rays using the Cobb method.

Cobb method: (fig 5.2)

1) Draw horizontal lines from the vertebral bodies of the extreme ends of the curve.
2) Draw perpendicular lines from these horizontal lines and measure the acute (Cobb) angle.

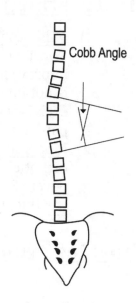

Fig 5.2: *Cobb Angle shown measures the degree of scoliosis.*

IV. Severity of Scoliosis [1 p.468]

Severity	Cobb angle
Mild	$5^o - 15^o$
Moderate	$20^o - 45^o$
Severe	$>50^o$

Respiratory function is compromised if the thoracic curvature is $>50^o$. Cardiovascular function is compromised if the thoracic curvature is $>75^o$.

V. Causes of Scoliosis [1 p. 468]

1) <u>Idiopathic</u> – approximately 70-90% of all causes of scoliosis. Some patients may have a family history of scoliosis suggesting a genetic component.

2) <u>Congenital</u> – Second most common cause, most. Often due to a malformation of the vertebrae. These cases are most often progressive.

3) <u>Acquired</u> – examples include tumor, infection, osteomalacia, sciatic irritability, response to inflammation or irradiation, healed leg fracture, hip prosthesis, and psoas syndrome.

VI. <u>Treatment</u> [1 p.470]

1) <u>Mild Scoliosis</u> – Conservative management will consist of physical therapy, Konstancin exercises and OMT. The goal of conservative treatment is to improve flexibility and strengthen trunk and abdominal musculature. OMT is not intended to completely straighten scoliotic curves.[1 p. 470] Konstantin exercises is a series of specific exercises that some authors feel beneficial in patients with scoliotic postural decompensation.[7 p.339]

2) <u>Moderate Scoliosis</u> – in addition to the above, bracing with a spinal orthotic (Milwaukee or Boston brace) is often indicated.

3) <u>Severe Scoliosis</u> – Consider surgery and adjunctive measures including treatments listed for moderate scoliosis

<u>Short leg syndrome</u>

I. <u>Definition</u>

Condition in which there is anatomical or functional leg length discrepancy. *The clinically relevent element in this syndrome is an unlevel sacral base.*[1 p.463]

II. <u>Classifications</u>

1) <u>Anatomical leg length discrepancy</u> – one leg *anatomically* shorter than the other.
   - *Most common cause is a hip replacement.*

2) <u>Functional leg length discrepancy</u> – one leg *appears* shorter than the other.

III. <u>Signs and Symptoms</u>

Although each person with short leg syndrome will compensate differently, certain structural findings can be present. They are:[1 p.463-4, 598 7 p.344]

1) Sacral base unleveling - the sacral base will be lower on the side of the short leg.
2) Anterior innominate rotation on the side of the short leg.
3) Posterior innominate rotation on the side of the long leg.
4) Pelvic side shift to the long leg side
5) Lumbar spine will sidebend away and rotate toward the side of the short leg.
6) An anterior sacrum (or forward sacral torsion) on the side of the short leg.[1p.598] (for example, right short leg = anterior sacrum right = Left on Left torsion)
7) First the iliolumbar ligaments, then the Si ligaments may become stressed on the side of the short leg.

IV. <u>Treatment</u>[1 p.464, 7 p. 346]

1) OMT directed at the spine and lower extremities done to remove or decrease as much somatic dysfunction as possible. If a leg length discrepancy is still present and short leg syndrome is still suspected then:
2) Obtain standing postural x-rays to quantify differences in the heights of the femoral head. If femoral head difference is > 5mm then consider a heel lift.

V. <u>Heel Lift Guidelines</u>[1 p.465, 7 p.346]

<u>Goal</u> – The objective of lift therapy is to level the sacral base[20 p.424]

1) The heel lift should be applied to the side of the short leg.
2) The final lift height should be ½ - ¾ of the measured leg length discrepancy, unless there was a recent sudden cause of the discrepancy (i.e. hip fracture or hip prosthesis). In this case, lift the full amount that was lost.
3) The "fragile" (elderly, arthritic, osteoporotic, or having acute pain) patient should begin with a 1/16" (~1.5mm) heel lift and increase 1/16" every two weeks.
4) The "flexible" patient should begin with 1/8" (~3.2mm) heel lift and increase 1/8" every two weeks
5) A maximum of ¼" may be applied to the inside of the shoe. If > ¼" is needed then this must be applied to the outside of the shoe.
6) Maximum heel lift possible = ½". If more height is needed, an ipsilateral anterior sole lift extending from heel to toe should be used in order to keep the pelvis from rotating to the opposite side.

Chapter 5 Review Questions

1. A scoliotic patient presents with right upper back pain. Structural examination reveals a type I dysfunction from T3-T8 and a prominent kyphosis. The right scapula is posterior. Upon forward flexion there is paraspinal muscle prominence on the right upper thoracic area. What spinal motion pattern would you suspect in this scenario?

    A. extended and rotated left freely
    B. sidebent left and rotated left freely at the apex segment only
    C. sidebent left and rotated right freely
    D. sidebent right and rotated left freely
    E. sidebent right and rotated right freely at the apex segment only

2. A patient has a type I curvature from T6-T12, convex left. The apex of the segment is T9. You would expect the thoracic spine to

    A. freely rotate left
    B. freely translate right
    C. maximally rotate right at the apex segment
    D. maximally sidebend left at the apex segment
    E. rotate and sidebend to the same direction

3. A young adult presents with low back pain and measurements reveal an anatomic short leg on the right side. This is most associated with

    A. anatomic landmarks (PSIS, iliac crest, greater trochanter) low on the left
    B. compensatory lumbar curve convex right
    C. pelvic rotation right due to right on right forward torsion
    D. pelvic side shift toward the right
    E. tender iliolumbar ligament on the left

Questions 4-6 refer to the following:

A 12-year-old female presents for routine follow-up for her chronic thoracic scoliosis. She has minimal symptoms but is cosmetically not pleased with her appearance. Structural examination reveals a small paravertebral hump on the right that improves with right sidebending.

4. A plain film radiograph is obtained and the Cobb angle of 12 degrees is measured which is stable from prior imaging. This angle represents the intersection of

    A. lines drawn parallel to the flexed or extended position of the superior vertebra and inferior vertebra in the coronal plane
    B. lines drawn parallel to the flexed or extended position of the superior vertebra and inferior vertebra in the sagittal plane
    C. tangential lines drawn from the end plate of the superior vertebra and the end plate of the inferior vertebra in the coronal plane
    D. tangential lines drawn from the superior end plate of the superior vertebra and the inferior end plate of the inferior vertebra in the sagittal plane
    E. tangential lines drawn from either the superior end plate of the superior vertebra or inferior end plate of the inferior vertebra and midline of the apex vertebra in the sagittal plane

5. Prognosis and management options are discussed. Surgery for scoliosis is most likely to have favorable results in which of the following cases?

    A. in a patient whose curve has progressed 10 degrees within 1 year
    B. in a patient whose curve has progressed after bracing and is causing respiratory compromise
    C. in a patient with a Cobb angle of 35 degrees
    D. in a patient with idiopathic scoliosis with a Cobb angle of 30 degrees
    E. in a skeletally mature patient with a Cobb angle of 40 degrees

6. Which of the following is the most appropriate management in this patient?

    A. heel lift therapy
    B. OMT, physical therapy and patient/family education
    C. observation with monthly radiography
    D. spinal fusion with harrington rods
    E. spinal orthotics

Questions 7-8 refer to the following:
    An elderly patient presents for a general wellness visit without complaints. Structural examination reveals a group curve in the thoracic region.

7. Which of the following is most associated with this segment's spinal mechanics?

    A. maximum rotation at the base of the curve
    B. rotation and sidebending directed toward the concavity
    C. rotation into the concavity when sidebending is introduced
    D. sidebending into the concavity with rotation into the convexity
    E. the posterior component is on the side of the concavity

8. The most likely cause in this patient is

    A. Idiopathic
    B. Cerebral palsy
    C. Congenital malformation of the vertebrae
    D. Psoas syndrome
    E. Inflammatory response

Questions 9-11 refer to the following:
   A 15-year-old female presents for routine follow-up for idiopathic scoliosis. History
   is significant for exertional dyspnea with an associated decreased respiratory
   excursion. Structural examination is significant for obvious paravertebral humping
   on the right. A comprehensive evaluation for cardiovascular disease is
   unremarkable; however pulmonary function testing is abnormal.

9. Which of the following is most associated with this patient's condition?

    A. a Cobb angle measuring 52 degrees
    B. a Cobb angle measuring 77 degrees
    C. scoliosis secondary to Duchenne muscular dystrophy
    D. scoliosis secondary to osteomalacia
    E. scoliosis secondary to a hemivertebrae

10. The paravertebral hump seen during structural examination is the result of

    A. contralateral paravertebral muscular atrophy
    B. displacement of the ribs on the side of the concavity of the spinal curve due to
       vertebral rotation
    C. ipsilateral paravertebral muscular hypertrophy
    D. prominence of the transverse processes on the side of the concavity of the
       spinal curve
    E. spinal rotation

11. The most likely diagnosis is

    A. dextroscoliosis with segment rotated left, sidebent right
    B. dextroscoliosis with segment rotated right, sidebent left
    C. levoscoliosis with segment rotated left, sidebent right
    D. levoscoliosis with segment rotated right, sidebent left
    E. levoscoliosis with segment rotated right, sidebent right

Questions ;12-13 refer to the following:

A 65-year-old female presents with acute low back pain. Observation reveals she has a frail body habitus with a wide-based, antalgic gait. Physical examination reveals a leg length discrepancy of 5/8th inches. A postural radiographic series is obtained and reveals the right femoral head is 1/2 inch cephalad when compared to the left.

12. The most appropriate initial management is

    A. Anterior (sole) lift of 1/4 inch and recheck postural study before attempting heel lifts
    B. Shoe lift of 1/4 inches and follow-up in 8 weeks
    C. Heel lift of 1/16 inch and follow up in 2 weeks
    D. Heel lift of 1/8 inch and increased 1/8 inches every 4 weeks until the pain has resolved
    E. Shoe lift of 5/8 inches and follow-up in two weeks

13. The most valid objective for heel lift therapy is to

    A. correct iliac crest difference
    B. correct leg length difference
    C. level the sacral base
    D. treat a primary lumbar curve
    E. treat a primary thoracic curve

Questions 14-15 refer to the following:

A 75-year-old male complains of persistent buttock pain despite right total hip arthroplasty. Standing palpatory examination reveals the iliac crest and greater trochanter to be inferior on the left. Postural radiographic studies reveal an unlevel sacral base that is inferior on the left.

14. The most likely cause of this patient's leg length discrepancy is

    A. hip dislocation
    B. osteoarthritis of the left hip
    C. left protrusio acetabuli
    D. scoliosis
    E. total hip replacement

15. The structural exam finding most associated with this presentation is

    A. compensatory spinal curve convex right
    B. left pelvic rotation
    C. pelvic side shift to the right
    D. posterior innominate on the left
    E. anterior sacrum right

Explanations

1. Answer: **C**

   This patient has a dextroscoliosis (convex right) from T3-T8 that is neutral, rotated right, sidebent left (T3-8 NR_RS_L) meaning the region will move more freely in those directions. The right rotation causes the paraspinal prominence noted in the questions stem. In the thoracic spine, the scapula protrudes posteriorly due to the paraspinal prominence. The apex will exhibit maximal rotation but is not the only segment that will sidebend left and rotate right, the entire group dysfunction will move in that direction.

2. Answer: **A**

   The patient has a levoscoliosis (convex left) from T6-T12 that is neutral, rotated left, sidebent right (T6-T12 NR_LS_R meaning the region will move more freely in those directions. Right translation is the same as left sidebending, which will be restricted in this patient. The apex of the curve will maximally rotate left.

3. Answer: **B**

   The lumbar spine will sidebend away (convex toward) and rotate toward the side of the short leg. The side of the short leg may also have an ipsilateral tender iliolumbar ligament, lower anatomic landmarks on the short side, and ipsilateral deep sacral sulcus due to an anterior sacrum or forward torsion (in this case L-on-L). The pelvic side shift will be positive toward the longer leg.

4. Answer: **C**

   The Cobb angle is the angle formed between the intersection of tangential lines drawn from the endplate of the top vertebra of the segment and the end-plate of the bottom vertebra of the segment. This is done in the coronal plane relative to the patient's degree of sidebending. The intersection of perpendicular lines drawn from these tangential lines will also provide the same angle measured as the tangential lines drawn from the vertebrae.

5. Answer: **B**

   Surgery is generally reserved for those with severe, progressive scoliosis involving Cobb angles ≥ 50 degrees in order to prevent respiratory or cardiovascular compromise. Those with Cobb angles ≥ 40-45 degrees can be considered for surgery to prevent progression.

6. Answer: **B**

This patient has mild scoliosis. While observation alone may be appropriate in this setting, typically those with Cobb angles 10-30 degrees benefit from radiography every 6 months until skeletally mature or until the angle ceases to progress. Monthly radiography is inappropriate and would not likely modify management in this patient. For mild scoliotic curves, OMT, physical therapy, and patient/family education is indicated. [1 p.470] Bracing (spinal orthotics) is reserved for Cobb angles >20 degrees (moderate scoliosis).

7. Answer: **D**

Group curves follow Fryette type I mechanics with rotation and sidebending to opposite sides. The concavity represents the direction toward sidebending while the convexity is the side away from sidebending. The posterior component (transverse process) will be appreciated on the side of the rotating segment, which is the convexity for group curves. Maximum rotation is at the apex of the curve.

8. Answer: **A**

The most common cause of scoliosis is idiopathic, and represents 70-90% of cases. Osteopathic physicians believe some of these may be explained as being compensatory curves due to an unlevel sacral or cranial base. [1 p.468] Cerebral palsy, congenital malformation, psoas syndrome, and reaction to inflammatory changes are all associated with an acquired cause of scoliosis.

9. Answer: **A**

This item is asking what type or severity of scoliosis is associated with respiratory compromise but not cardiovascular disease. The patient in question has respiratory compromise evident by the decreased ability to fully inspire, limiting exertional capacity and abnormal pulmonary function tests. Individuals with Cobb angles greater than 50 degrees typically have signs of respiratory compromise while those with angles greater than 75 degrees may have signs of cardiovascular compromise. Duchenne muscular dystrophy is an x-lined recessive condition that only affects males (patient is female). Scoliosis secondary to osteomalacia is an acquired scoliosis; this is incorrect since the patient has idiopathic scoliosis. Scoliosis secondary to a hemivertebrae is a congenital cause of scoliosis.

10. Answer: **E**

The paravertebral hump seen in scoliotic patients is due to displacement of the ribs on the side of the convexity secondary to spinal rotation.

11. Answer: **B**

Scoliotic curves are named for the side of convexity which is opposite to the sidebending side. Group curves follow Fryette type I mechanics and rotate and sidebend in opposite directions. The right-sided paravertebral humping is due to right vertebral rotation. Therefore, the segment is also sidebent left and termed a dextroscoliosis.

12. Answer: **C**

The initial amount of lift selected is rarely the full amount needed unless there was a sudden loss of leg length and the patient had a level sacral base prior to the loss. Since this patient is elderly and presenting with acute pain it is best to begin with a 1/16 inch heel lift and reevaluate in 2 weeks. If this patient was not 'fragile' (e.g., arthritic, osteoporotic, elderly) then a 1/8 inch lift with reevaluation in 2 weeks could be considered. Anterior (sole) lifts cause the pelvis to rotate posteriorly in the horizontal plane; they are prescribed for those with pelvic rotation >1 cm (~3/8th inch). Those with sacral base unleveling and pelvic rotation are treated simultaneously with 1/8 inch incremental changes in anterior and heel lifts every 2 weeks.

13. Answer: **C**

The objective of lift therapy is functional balance of the sacral base. Leveling the sacra base through heel lift therapy is successful in reducing and eliminating chronic musculoskeletal pain.[20 p.424]

14. Answer: **E**

The most common cause of an anatomically short leg is a total hip replacement. Pelvic (sacral) unleveling is likely the cause of the persistent buttock pain. The sacrum should be balanced using OMT and heel lift therapy, then re-evaluated for other possible causes of persistent buttock pain. Protrusio acetabuli is an uncommon pathologic displacement of the femoral head medial to the ischioilial line.

15. Answer: **C**

This patient has a short leg on the left side. This is associated with a pelvic shift to the long leg (right), anterior innominate rotation on the short leg, posterior innominate rotation on the long leg, lumbar spine sidebent right (i.e. levoscoliosis, convexity left) and anterior sacrum (forward sacral torsion) on left.

<h1>SACRUM & INNOMINATES 6</h1>

<h2>I. <u>Anatomy</u></h2>

<h3>A. <u>Bones and bony landmarks</u></h3>

1. <u>Innominate</u>: The innominate is composed of three fused bones, the ilium, the ischium and pubis bones.

2. <u>Sacrum</u>: The sacrum is composed of five fused vertebrae. The anterior portion of the first segment (S1) is referred to as the *sacral promontory*. The *sacral base* is the top (most cephalad) part of the sacrum. In somatic dysfunctions, the sacral base can be recorded as shallow (or posterior) or deep (or anterior). The *sacral apex* is the bottom part of the sacrum, which articulates with the coccyx. The *sacral sulci* are located on the superior lateral part of the sacrum (see figure 6.1). They are recorded as posterior (or shallow) or anterior (or deep) in somatic dysfunctions. The

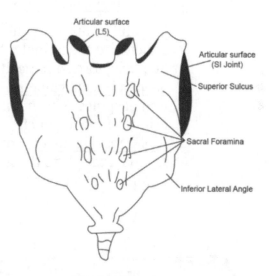

Fig 6.1: *The sacrum*

inferior lateral angles (ILA's) of the sacrum are located at the inferior lateral part of the sacrum. They are recorded as shallow (or posterior), deep (or anterior), superior or inferior in somatic dysfunctions.

<u>NOTE</u>: In some osteopathic schools, the right sacral sulcus is referred to as the right sacral base. The left sacral sulcus is referred to as the left sacral base. In somatic dysfunctions, the right (or left) sacral base could be anterior or posterior.

B. Articulations

The innominates articulate with the femur at the acetabulum and the sacrum at the SI joint The pubic bones articulate with each other at the pubic symphysis. The SI joint is an inverted "L" shaped joint with upper and lower arms converging anteriorly. These two arms join at S2. Somatic dysfunction may occur in one or both arms of the SI joint. [8 p. 619]

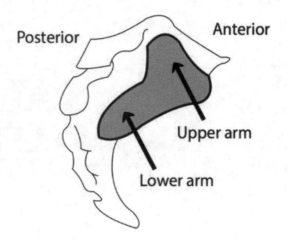

Fig 6.2: The SI joint is an inverted "L" joint with the 2 arms converging anteriorly.

C. Ligaments

Pelvic ligaments can be categorized into true or accessory pelvic ligaments.[7p.406]

1. True pelvic ligaments (Sacroiliac ligaments)
   Anterior, posterior and interosseous sacroiliac ligaments surround and help stabilize the SI joint.

2. Accessory pelvic ligaments

   a. Sacrotuberous ligament – originates at the inferior lateral angle and attaches to the ischial tuberosity. Testing the tension of this ligament can help diagnose somatic dysfunction of the innominate or sacrum.[7 p.407]
   b. Sacrospinous ligament – originates at the sacrum and attaches to the ischial spines. *This ligament divides this region, creating the greater and lesser sciatic foramen*
   c. Iliolumbar ligament – originates from the transverse processes of L4 and L5 and attaches to the medial side of the iliac crest. *It is often the first ligament to become painful in lumbosacral decompensation.*[7 p.407]

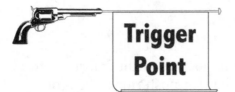

The Sacrospinous ligament divides the greater and lesser sciatic foramen.

D. Muscles
Pelvic muscles can be categorized into **primary** and **secondary** muscles.[61 p.578, 28 p.408]

1. Primary pelvic muscles – These muscles make up the *pelvic diaphragm.*[1 p.578]

   a. Levator ani
   b. Coccygeus muscles
      Clinical importance – Levator ani and the coccygeus muscles work in synchrony with the abdomimal diaphragm to move lymphatic fluid from the pelvis and perineal tissues. [1 p.580]

2. Secondary pelvic muscles – These muscles have partial attachments to the pelvis. There are several secondary pelvic muscles. Spasm of these muscles can lead to sacral and innominate dysfunction. [1 p.579]

E. Nerves The nervous system can influence the pelvic girdle through one of four areas. These are: [1 p.581]

1. Lumbar plexus - ventral rami of T12-L4
2. Sacral plexus
3. Coccygeal plexus
4. Autonomic nerves of the pelvis

II. Sacral and innominate mechanics

A. Innominates (see Fig. 6.3)

Physiologically, the innominates rotate about an inferior transverse axis of the sacrum during the walking cycle (dotted line in figure 6.3). The axis is located in the posterior-inferior portion of the inferior limb of the SI joint. It is also the axis which an innominate anterior or innominate posterior somatic dysfunction occur.

B. Sacrum

1. **Four types of sacral motion** (see Fig. 6.3)

   a. Respiratory motion – *Motion occurs about the superior transverse axis of the sacrum.* It is located at approximately S2 posterior to the SI joint.[1 p.583] During inhalation, the sacral base will move posterior. During exhalation, the sacral base will move anterior. [1 p.585]

b. <u>Inherent (craniosacral) motion</u> – *Motion occurs about the superior transverse axis of the sacrum (same axis for respiratory motion). During craniosacral flexion, the sacral base rotates posteriorly or* **counternutates**. *During craniosacral extension, the sacral base rotates anteriorly or* **nutates**.[1 p.585]

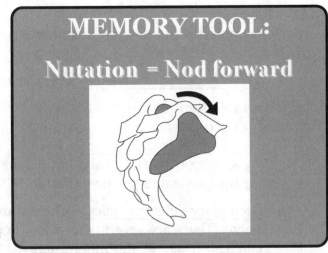

MEMORY TOOL:

Nutation = Nod forward

c. <u>Postural motion</u> – *Motion occurs about the middle transverse axis of the sacrum.* It is located at the anterior convexity of the upper and lower limbs of the SI joint. As a person begins to bend forward, the sacral base moves anteriorly. At terminal flexion, the sacrotuberous ligaments become taut and the sacral base will move posteriorly.[1 p.585, 7 p.176]

d. <u>Dynamic motion</u> – *Motion that occurs during ambulation.* As weight bearing shifts from one side to the other while walking, the sacrum engages two sacral oblique axes. *Weight bearing on the left leg (stepping forward with the right leg) will cause a left sacral axis to be engaged.* The opposite is true for weight bearing on the right leg.[1 p. 585]

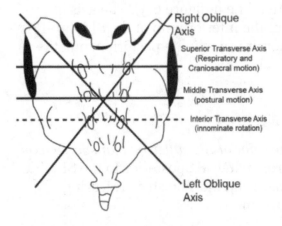

Fig 6.3: *Physiologic axes of the sacrum and innominate: Respiratory and craniosacral motions occurs about the superior transverse axis. Postural motion occurs about the middle transverse axis. Dynamic motion occurs about a left or right oblique axes. Innominate rotation occurs about an inferior transverse axis.*

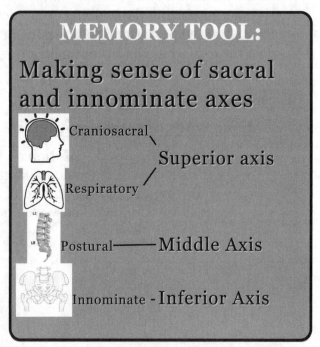

MEMORY TOOL:

Making sense of sacral and innominate axes

Craniosacral
Superior axis
Respiratory
Postural——Middle Axis
Innominate - Inferior Axis

MEMORY TOOL:

Physiologic axes of the sacrum and innominates = "D.R.I.P."

D = dynamic

R = respiratory

I = inherent/innominate

P = postural

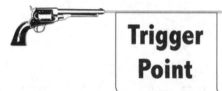

Trigger Point

Know the physiologic motion and axes of the sacrum.

III. Somatic dysfunctions of the innominates

A. Innominate dysfunction (Remember, the side of the positive standing flexion test is the side of the dysfunction.)

1. Anterior innominate rotation

One innominate will rotate anteriorly compared to the other. Rotation occurs about the inferior transverse axis of the sacrum.

Etiology: tight quadriceps

Static findings:[1 p.588, 10 p.219]

ASIS more inferior ipsilaterally

PSIS more superior ipsilaterally

Tissue texture changes at the ipsilateral ILA of sacrum

Iliolumbar ligament tenderness

Dynamic findings:[1 p.588, 10 p.219, 21 p.215]

Positive standing flexion test ipsilaterally

Posterior innominate rotation is restricted ipsilaterally

Postive ASIS compression test ipsilaterally

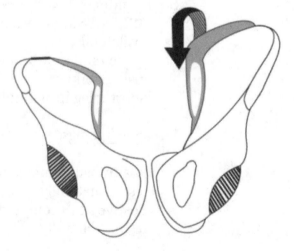

Fig. 6.4: *Left innominate anterior*

2. <u>Posterior innominate rotation</u>

One innominate will rotate posteriorly compared to the other. Rotation occurs about the inferior transverse axis of the sacrum.

<u>Etiology:</u> tight hamstrings
<u>Static findings:</u> [8 p.617, 10 p.214]

    ASIS more superior ipsilaterally.
    PSIS more inferior ipsilaterally.
    Inguinal tenderness
    Tissue texture changes at the ipsilateral sacral sulcus.

<u>Dynamic findings:</u> [1 p.588, 10 p.214, 21 p.215]

    Positive standing flexion test ipsilaterally
    ASIS restricted to compression ipsilaterally

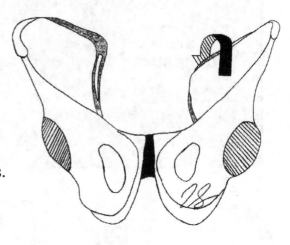

Fig. 6.5:   *Left innominate posterior*

3. <u>Superior innominate shear (subluxation)</u>[1] a.k.a. <u>innominate upslip</u>[10]

One innominate will slip superiorly compared to the other.

<u>Etiology:</u> It can be due to a fall on the ipsilateral buttock or a mis-step

<u>Static findings:</u> [1 p.588, 10 p.223, 21 p.215]

    ASIS & PSIS more superior ipsilaterally
    Pubic rami may be superior ipsilaterally
    Shorter leg ipsilaterally

<u>Dynamic findings:</u> [1 p.588, 10 p.223, 21 p.215]

    Positive standing flexion test ipsilaterally
    Postive ASIS compression test ipsilaterally

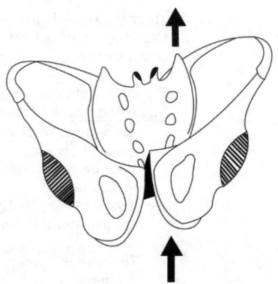

Fig. 6.6:   *Left superior innominate shear*

4. <u>Inferior innominate shear (subluxation) [1]a.k.a. innominate downslip[33]</u>

One innominate will slip inferiorly compared to the other.

<u>Static findings:</u>[1 p.588, 21 p.215]
> ASIS & PSIS more inferior ipsilaterally
> Pubic rami may be inferior ipsilaterally
> Longer leg ipsilaterally

<u>Dynamic findings:</u> [1 p.588, 21 p.215]
> Positive standing flexion test ipsilaterally
> Postive ASIS compression test ipsilaterally

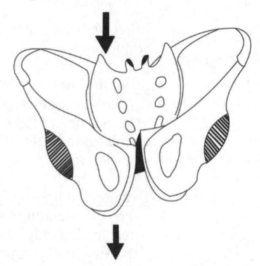

Fig. 6.7: *Right inferior innominate shear*

5. <u>Superior pubic shear</u>

A condition where one pubic bone is displaced superiorly compared to the other.

<u>Etiology:</u> trauma or a tight rectus abdominus muscle

<u>Static findings:</u>[1 p.588, 10 p.185]
> ASIS's appear to be level
> PSIS's appear to be level
> Pubic bone superior ipsilaterally

<u>Dynamic findings:</u>[1 p.588, 10 p.185]
> Positive standing flexion test ipsilaterally
> Postive ASIS compression test ipsilaterally

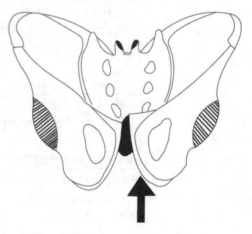

Fig. 6.8: *Left superior pubic shear*

6. **Inferior pubic shear**

A condition where one pubic bone is displaced inferiorly compared to the other.

<u>Etiology</u>: trauma or tight adductors

<u>Static findings</u>:[1 p.588, 10 p.187]
ASIS's appear to be level
PSIS's appear to be level
Pubic bone inferiorly ipsilaterally.

<u>Dynamic findings</u>:[1 p.588, 10 p.187]
Positive standing flexion test ipsilaterally
Postive ASIS compression test ipsilaterally

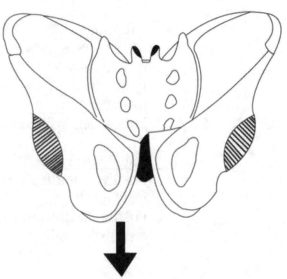

Fig. 6.9: *Right inferior pubic shear*

7. **Innominate inflares**

A condition where the innominate will rotate medially around a vertical axis. Inflares tend to occur simultaneously with anterior innominate rotation.[1 p.589]

<u>Static findings</u>:[10 p.224]
ASIS more medial ipsilaterally. Therefore the distance between the ASIS and umbilicus is less than that of the contralateral side.
Ischial tuberosity more lateral ipsilaterally.

<u>Dynamic findings</u>:[10 p.224]
Positive standing flexion test ipsilaterally.
Postive ASIS compression test ipsilaterally.

8. **Innominate outflare**

A condition where the innominate will rotate laterally around a vertical axis. Outflares tend to occur simultaneously with posterior innominate rotation. [1 p.589]

<u>Static findings</u>:[10 p.224]
ASIS more lateral ipsilaterally. Therefore the distance between the ASIS and umbilicus is more than that of the contralateral side.
Ischial tuberosity more medial ipsilaterally.

<u>Dynamic findings</u>:[10 p.224]
Positive standing flexion test ipsilaterally.
Postive ASIS compression test ipsilaterally

IV. Somatic dysfunctions of the Sacrum

There are two models to describe sacral dysfunction.

1. In 1938, Strachan *described sacral movements in relation to the ilium.* Strachan noted two sacral somatic dysfunctions.

   a. Anterior sacrum – the left or right sacral base will rotate **forward** and sidebend to the opposite side of rotation. The movement of the sacrum is about an oblique axis and the findings are very similar to a forward sacral torsion (see below).

   b. Posterior sacrum – the left or right sacral base will rotate **backward** and sidebend to the opposite of the rotation. The movement of the sacrum is about an oblique axis and the findings are very similar to a backward sacral torsion (see below).

2. In 1958, Mitchell *described sacral motion in relation to L5.* According to Mitchell, three sacral somatic dysfunctions are possible. They are:
   a. Sacral torsions/sacral rotation on an oblique axis
   b. Sacral shears (unilateral sacral flexions/extensions)
   c. Bilateral sacral flexions/extensions

A. Sacral Torsions

1. Definition – *Sacral rotation about an oblique axis along with somatic dysfunction at L5.* The oblique axis will run through the superior sulcus ipsilaterally, diagonally across the sacrum and through the contralateral ILA.

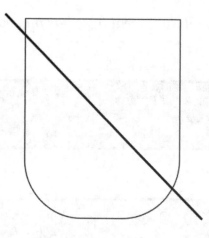

Fig. 6.10: *Posterior view of the sacrum with a left oblique axis. The axis is named for the side of the superior pole it runs through.*

2. Sacral torsion rules – Due to lumbosacral biomechanics, if a sacral torsion is present, certain reproducible L5 and seated flexion test findings are produced. These "Rules" can be summarized as follows:

Sacral Torsion Rules:

a. **Rule #1**: *When L5 is sidebent, a sacral oblique axis is engaged on the same side as the sidebending.*

b. **Rule #2**: *When L5 is rotated, the sacrum rotates the opposite way on an oblique axis.*

c. **Rule #3**: *The seated flexion test is found on the opposite side of the oblique axis.*

Putting the rules together:

If L5 is FR_RS_R:

There will be a positive seated flexion test on the left.

The sacrum will be rotated to the left on a right oblique axis or L on R.

If L5 (or a group dysfunction of the lower lumbar region) is NS_LR_R:

There will be a positive seated flexion test on the right.

The sacrum will be rotated to the left on a left oblique axis or L on L.

3. Palpatory model for sacral torsions [10]

Springing over sacral landmarks in sacral torsions

– *Springing (motion) present over the part of the sacrum that moved anterior.*

– *Springing (motion) restricted over the part of the sacrum that moved posterior*

– *Springing (motion) restricted over the poles that make up the oblique axis*

– *Lumbosacral spring test is positive if the sacral base has moved posterior.*

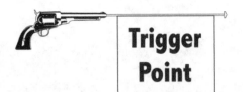

Trigger Point

Know the rules of L5 on the sacrum.

MEMORY TOOL:

Torsion = twisting of two articulating structures (L5 and the Sacrum) in *opposite* directions.

In sacral torsions, L5 will always rotate in the *opposite* direction of the sacrum.

1. **Forward sacral torsion**
    In a forward sacral torsion, rotation is on the same side of the axis.

    Two dysfunctions are possible:

    a. Left rotation on a left oblique axis (L on L):
        left rotation occurs as the right superior sulcus
        moves anterior while the left ILA moves
        posterior.

        <u>Static findings:</u>[1 p.594, 10 p.203]
            Right sulcus deeper.
            Left ILA posterior
            Lumbar curve convex to the right.

        <u>Dynamic findings:</u>[1 p.594, 2 p.320, 10 p.203]
            Positive seated flexion test on the RIGHT.
            Motion (springing) at the right base is present.
            Motion (springing) at the left ILA is restricted.
            Motion (springing) at the poles of the left oblique axis (left sulcus and
            right ILA) is restricted.
            Negative lumbosacral spring test
            L5 will be sidebent left rotated right ($NS_L R_R$).

    b. <u>Right rotation on a right oblique axis (R on R)</u>: right rotation occurs as
        the left superior sulcus moves anterior, while the right ILA moves
        posterior.

        <u>Static findings:</u>[1 p.594, 10 p.203]
            Left sulcus deeper.
            Right ILA posterior and slightly inferior.
            Lumbar curve convex to the left.

        <u>Dynamic findings:</u>[1 p.594, 2 p.320, 10 p.203]
            Positive seated flexion test on the LEFT.
            Motion (springing) at the left base is present.
            Motion (springing) at the right ILA is
            restricted.
            Motion (springing) at the poles of the right
            oblique axis (right sulcus and left ILA) is
            restricted.
            Negative lumbosacral spring test
            L5 will be sidebent right, rotated left ($NS_R R_L$).

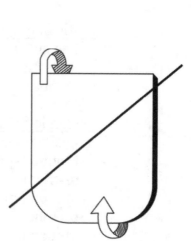

2. Backward sacral torsion

In a backward sacral torsion, rotation is on the opposite side of the axis.

Two dysfunctions are possible:

a. <u>Right rotation on a left oblique axis (R on L)</u>: right rotation occurs as the right superior sulcus moves posterior, and the left ILA moves anterior.

<u>Static findings:</u>[1 p.594, 10 p. 208]
> Right sulcus shallow.
> Left ILA anterior and slightly superior.
> Lumbar curve convex to the right.

<u>Dynamic findings:</u>[1 p.594, 2 p.320, 10 p.203]

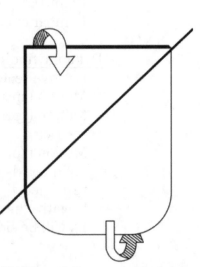

> Positive seated flexion test on the RIGHT.
> Motion (springing) at the right base is restricted.
> Motion (springing) at the left ILA is present.
> Motion (springing) at the poles of the left oblique axis (left sulcus and right ILA) is restricted.
> Positive lumbosacral spring test.
> Positive backward bending test.
> L5 will be flexed or extended (nonneutral), sidebent left, rotated left (NNR_LS_L).

b. <u>Left rotation on a right oblique axis (L on R)</u>: left rotation occurs as the left superior sulcus moves posterior, and the right ILA moves anterior.

<u>Static findings:</u>[1 p.594, 10 p. 208]
> Left sulcus shallow.
> Right ILA anterior and slightly superior.
> Lumbar curve convex to the left.

<u>Dynamic findings:</u>[1 p.594, 2 p 320, 10 p.203]

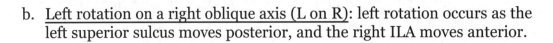

> Positive seated flexion test on the LEFT.
> Motion (springing) at the left base is restricted.
> Motion (springing) at the right ILA is present.
> Motion (springing) at the poles of the right oblique axis (right sulcus and left ILA) is restricted.
> Positive lumbosacral spring test.
> Positive backward bending test.
> L5 will be flexed or extended (nonneutral), sidebent right, rotated right (NNR_RS_R).

3. Bilateral sacral flexion and extension

a. <u>Bilateral sacral flexion (sacral base anterior)</u>

In this somatic dysfunction, the entire sacral base moves anterior about a middle transverse axis.[1 p.595, 7 p.402]

<u>Static findings:</u>[1 p.594, 10 p.191]
Right and left sulci deep.
ILA's shallow bilaterally.
Increased lumbar curve.

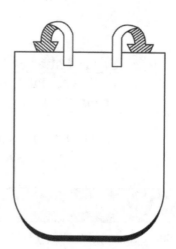

<u>Dynamic findings:</u>[1 p.594, 2 p 320, 10 p.191]
FALSE negative seated flexion test.
  <u>NOTE</u>: since both SI joints are restricted in this dysfunction, asymmetry cannot be appreciated, resulting in a false negative seated and standing flexion tests.
Motion (springing) at both sulci (base) is present.
Motion (springing) at both ILA's (apex) is restricted.
Negative lumbosacral spring test.

b. <u>Bilateral sacral extensions (sacral base posterior)</u>

In this somatic dysfunction, the entire sacral base moves posterior about a middle transverse axis.[1 p.595, 7 p.402]

<u>Static findings:</u>[1 p.594, 10 p.195]
Right and left sulci shallow.
ILA's deeper bilaterally.
Decreased lumbar curve.

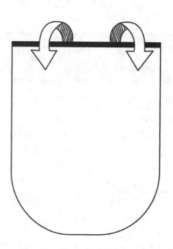

<u>Dynamic findings:</u>[1 p.594, 2 p 320, 10 p.195]
FALSE negative seated flexion test.
  NOTE: Since both SI joints are restricted in this dysfunction, asymmetry cannot be appreciated, resulting in a false negative seated and standing flexion tests.
Motion (springing) at both sulci (base) is restricted.
Motion (springing) at both ILA's (apex) is present.
Positive lumbosacral spring test.

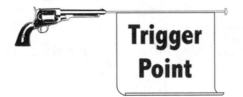

4. **Sacral shears (unilateral sacral flexion/extension) (USF/USE)**
In this somatic dysfunction, the sacrum will shift anteriorly or posteriorly around a transverse axis. [1 p.595]

   a. Unilateral sacral flexion on the right (USF_R) or left (USF_L).
   b. Unilateral sacral extension on the right (USE_R) or left (USE_L).

Left unilateral sacral flexion	Right unilateral sacral flexion

Static findings: [1 p.594, 10 p.211]
   Left sulcus deeper.
   Left ILA significantly inferior
   Left ILA slightly posterior.
	Static findings: [1 p.594, 10 p.211]
	   Right sulcus deeper.
	   Right ILA significantly inferior
	   Right ILA slightly posterior.

Dynamic findings: [1 p.594, 10 p.211]
   Positive seated flexion test on the left.
   Motion (springing) at the left sulcus is present.
   Motion (springing) at the left ILA is restricted.
	Dynamic findings: [1 p.594, 10 p.211]
	   Positive seated flexion test on the right.
	   Motion (springing) at the right sulcus is present.
	   Motion (springing) at the right ILA is restricted.

5. **Sacral margin posterior**

Left unilateral sacral extension	Right unilateral sacral extension

Static findings: [61 p.594, 33 p.213]
   Left sulcus shallow.
   Left ILA significantly superior.
   Left ILA slightly anterior.
	Static findings: [61 p.594, 33 p.213]
	   Right sulcus shallow.
	   Right ILA significantly superior.
	   Right ILA slightly anterior.

Dynamic findings: [61 p.594, 33 p.213]
   Positive seated flexion test on the left.
   Motion (springing) at the left sulcus is restricted.
   Motion (springing) at the left ILA is present
   Positive lumbosacral spring test.
   Positive backward bending test.
	Dynamic findings: [61 p.594, 33 p.213]
	   Positive seated flexion test on the right.
	   Motion (springing) at the right sulcus is restricted.
	   Motion (springing) at the right ILA is present.
	   Positive lumbosacral spring test.
	   Positive backward bending test.

Some authors do not recognize this as a true somatic dysfunction, hence there is controversy on whether it exists. However, it is mentioned here because this dysfunction is taught at some osteopathic institutions. In a **sacral margin posterior,** the sacrum rotates posteriorly about a mid-vertical or parasagittal vertical axis.[10 p.198]

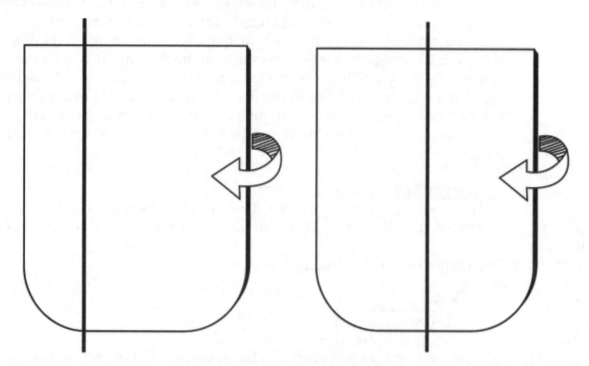

Fig. 6.11: *Right sacral margin about a parasagittal vertical axis.*

Fig. 6.12: *Right sacral margin about a mid-vertical axis.*

Right sacral margin *Vertical axis*	Right sacral margin *Parasagittal axis*
Static findings: Right sulci and right ILA shallow. Left sulci and left ILA deep	Static findings: Right sulci and right ILA shallow. Left sulci and left ILA normal
Dynamic findings: Motion (springing) on the right sulcus and right ILA is restricted. Motion (springing) on the left sulcus and left ILA is present.	Dynamic findings: Motion (springing) on the right sulcus and right ILA is restricted. Motion (springing) on the left sulcus and left ILA is present.

6. **Anterior and posterior sacrum** – These models were originally described by Strachan in 1938. These somatic dysfunctions describe sacral motion in relation to the ilium (as opposed to the Mitchell model which describes sacral motion in relation to L5). An anterior and posterior sacrum are oblique axis dysfunctions. [1 p.596] Strachan never commented on the sacrum in relation to L5 and therefore assessment of L5 requires a separate assessment.[1 p.591] These dysfunctions are very similar to forward or backward sacral torsion (without comment on L5). In an anterior sacrum left , the left sacral base rotates right (around an oblique axis - think right on right) and sidebends left compressing the upper arm of the SI joint. In a posterior sacrum left, the sacral base rotates left (around an oblique axis - think left on right) and sidebends right compressing the left lower arm of the SI joint). An anterior sacrum is considered a dysfunction in the upper arm of the SI joint, and a posterior sacrum is considered a dysfunction in the lower arm of the SI joint. [1 p.596]

a. Anterior Sacrum
In an anterior sacrum left, the left sacral sulcus has moved anterior around an oblique axis. *This is similar to a right on right sacral torsion.*

Anterior sacrum left findings:

Static findings:[1 p.596]
Left sulcus deeper.
Right ILA posterior
Tissue texture abnormality and tenderness in the deep sulcus
(because of dysfunction of the upper arm of the SI joint).

Dynamic findings: [1 p.596]
Positive seated flexion test on the LEFT.
Motion (springing) at the left base is present.
Motion (springing) at the right ILA is restricted.

b Posterior Sacrum
In an posterior sacrum left, the left sacral sulcus has moved posterior around an oblique axis. *This is similar to a left on right sacral torsion.*

Posterior sacrum left findings

<u>Static findings:</u>[1 p596]
Left sulcus shallow.
Right ILA anterior.
Tissue texture abnormality an tenderness in the shallow ILA.
(because of dysfunction of the lower arm of the SI joint)

<u>Dynamic findings:</u>[1 p.596]
Positive seated flexion test on the LEFT or RIGHT. (NOTE: in a posterior sacrum the seated flexion test can be positive on either side)
Motion (springing) at the left base is restricted.
Motion (springing) at the right ILA is present.

V. <u>Causes of Sacroiliac dysfunction</u>[1 p.598-99]

1. <u>Psoas</u> –
   Treatment of psoas dysfunction is the first step in treating SI dysfunction. The sacrum cannot function properly with excess psoas tension. Check for psoas tension and associated L1 or L2 dysfunctions. Failure to remove the psoas component will result in an SI dysfunction that recurs quickly

2. <u>Lumbar somatic dysfucntions</u>
   Lumbar dysfunctions, particularly flexed Type II dysfunctions can contribute to SI dysfunctions.

3. <u>Short leg syndrome/postural imbalances</u>
   A chronic anterior sacrum (or forward torsion) on the side of the short leg is a classic finding.

4. <u>Pelvic side shift (see chapter 18 for pelvic side shift test)</u>
   This is one mechanism of SI dysfunction associated with a contralateral tight psoas, a lumbar group curve (with convexity contralateral to the pelvic side shift) and or a short leg contralateral to the pelvic side shift.

5. <u>Simple traumatic sacral dysfunction</u>
   Typically two mechanisms:
   1. Slip and fall onto buttocks
   2. MVA where force of the impact travels through their brake leg into the pelvis.

6. <u>Pubic and pelvic floor dysfunctions</u>
   Improved pubic motion will allow the ilium to move freely
   Pubic dysfunction is associated with pelvic floor dysfunction

7. <u>Reflex causes</u>
   Viscerosomatic relfexes from the pelvis or unilateral sympathetic nervous system dysfunction are causes of SI joint pain.

8. <u>Cranial dysfunctions</u>
   Sacral motion or SI joint dysfunction can be due to strains or compression of the sphenobasilar symphysis (SBS)

9. <u>Lumbosacral instability</u>
   SI pain can be caused by orthopedic problems of L5-S1 (spondylolysis, spondylolithesis). Iliolumbar ligament tenderness is often associated with lumbosacral decompensation.

10. <u>Disc protrusions</u>
    Disc protrusions at L4 or L5 in early stages can radiate pain into the buttocks and is interpreted as SI joint pain. The sacrum my be restricted from secondary muscle hypertonicity.

VI. <u>Sequencing lumbar-sacrum-pelvis treatment</u>

It is generally accepted to treat the lumbar spine, psoas, iluim and pubes before treating the sacrum. [1] p.599

Chapter 6 Review Questions

1. A middle-aged adult present with right hip pain and is determined to have an anterior innominate rotation. This dysfunction occurs about the

    A. inferior transverse axis
    B. middle transverse axis
    C. oblique axis
    D. respiratory axis
    E. superior transverse axis

2. A 32-year-old female presents with sacroiliac pain that started 2 days ago after lifting her son. Structural examination reveals the following:

    • convex right lumbar curve
    • deep right sacral sulcus
    • L5 NSLRR
    • positive seated flexion test on the right
    • shallow left ILA

    The most likely diagnosis is

    A. left sacral rotation on a left oblique axis
    B. left sacral rotation on a right oblique axis
    C. right sacral rotation on a left oblique axis
    D. right sacral rotation on a right oblique axis
    E. unilateral sacral extension on the right

3. A 21-year-old male complains of gluteal pain of 2 days' duration. He states that the pain started after biking for several miles. History reveals he is obese and is not physically active. Structural examination reveals the sacral sulci are shallow with a positive lumbosacral spring test. The seated and standing flexion tests are both negative. The most likely diagnosis is a bilateral sacral

    A. flexion on a middle transverse axis
    B. flexion on a superior transverse axis
    C. flexion on an inferior transverse axis
    D. extension on a middle transverse axis
    E. extension on an inferior transverse axis

4. A 25-year-old male reports right-sided low back and sacroiliac pain 1 week after a prolonged period of sitting. Structural examination reveals tenderness over the right sacroiliac joint, a positivecseated flexion test on the right, the sacral sulcus on the right is anterior, and the right ILA is inferior and shallow. The most likely diagnosis is a unilateral sacral

   A. extension on the left about an oblique axis
   B. extension on the right about a transverse axis
   C. flexion on the left about an oblique axis
   D. flexion on the left about a transverse axis
   E. flexion on the right about a transverse axis

5. A 30-year-old runner presents with left-sided hip pain that started yesterday after a 5 mile run. It is sharp but does not radiate into the lower extremities. Structural examination reveals a positive standing flexion test on the left, the right ASIS is superior, the right PSIS is inferior, and the right leg is shorter. The most likely diagnosis is

   A. left anterior innominate
   B. left posterior innominate
   C. right posterior innominate
   D. unilateral sacral extension on the left
   E. unilateral sacral flexion on the left

6. A 40-year-old with low back pain has a deep sacral sulcus on the right. Which of the following is most consistent with this finding?

   A. right sacral rotation on a left oblique axis
   B. right sacral rotation on a right oblique axis
   C. unilateral sacral extension on the right
   D. unilateral sacral flexion on the left
   E. unilateral sacral flexion on the right

7. A 32-year-old female presents with sacroiliac pain that started 2 days ago after picking up her 3-year-old son. Examination reveals a positive seated flexion test on the right, L5 NSLRR, a shallow left ILA, deep right superior sulcus, and lumbar curve that is convex to the right. The most likely diagnosis is a

   A. left sacral rotation on a left oblique axis
   B. left sacral rotation on a right oblique axis
   C. right sacral rotation on a left oblique axis
   D. right sacral rotation on a right oblique axis
   E. unilateral sacral extension on the right

8. A 20-year-old male presents with low back pain following a fall onto a concrete floor. History reveals episodic aching of the lumbar region prior to the fall. Structural examination in the prone position reveals a deep sacral sulcus on the left, a posterior/inferior ILA on the right, and a lumbosacral junction that springs freely upon compression. The most likely diagnosis is a

    A. backward sacral torsion on a left oblique axis
    B. bilateral sacral extension
    C. forward sacral torsion on a left oblique axis
    D. forward sacral torsion on a right oblique axis
    E. left unilateral sacral flexion

9. A patient has a sacral torsion that resulted in a right anterior sacral base and a negative lumbosacral spring test. Structural examination will most likely reveal an L5 that is

    A. ER_RS_L
    B. FR_LS_L
    C. FR_RS_L
    D. NS_LR_R
    E. NS_RR_L

10. A 46-year-old male presents to your office complaining of chronic lumbosacral pain. There is a negative standing flexion test and a positive seated flexion test. Structural examination reveals a deep sacral sulcus on the left, posterior/inferior ILA on the right, and the lumbosacral junction springs freely upon compression. The most likely diagnosis is

    A. left sacral rotation on a left oblique axis
    B. left sacral rotation on a right oblique axis
    C. right sacral rotation on a left oblique axis
    D. right sacral rotation on a right oblique axis
    E. right sacral shear

11. In a patient with acute onset of low back pain, structural examination reveals a positive seated flexion test on the right. The left sacral base is anterior when compared to the right. The spring test is positive. What is the most likely sacral diagnosis?

    A. extended sacral base
    B. left sacral rotation on a right oblique axis
    C. right sacral rotation on a left oblique axis
    D. right sacral rotation on a right oblique axis
    E. right unilateral sacral flexion

Questions 12-14 refer to the following
    A 20-year-old presents for a general wellness visit without complaints. A comprehensive structural examination is performed.

12. The examiner locates and assesses the inferior lateral angles. These are best described as

    A. a general anatomic area at the lateral aspect of S4-S5
    B. the angle between the sacrospinous and sacrotuberous ligament at their attachment to the sacrum
    C. the curvature created by pseudoarthrosis between the coccyx and sacrum
    D. the long lower arm of the sacral "L-shaped" facet
    E. the lower half of either oblique axis

13. The sacrum is motion tested and an anteriorly-directed force is applied over the right inferior lateral angle. Which of the following most appropriately describes the expected findings with this motion?

    A. left sacral base will move posteriorly
    B. left sacral sulcus will move anteriorly
    C. sacrum will move about a left oblique axis
    D. sacrum will move about a purely vertical axis
    E. right ILA will move posteriorly

14. Which of the following is most accurate regarding the normal physiologic motion of the sacrum?

    A. during craniosacral flexion the sacral base will move posterior about a middle transverse axis
    B. during exhalation the sacral base will move posterior about an inferior transverse axis
    C. during inhalation the sacral base will move anterior about a superior axis
    D. during postural flexion the sacral base will move anterior about a superior transverse axis
    E. during swing phase of the right lower extremity the sacrum moves about a left oblique axis

Questions 15-16 refer to the following
    A 40-year-old presents with buttocks pain of 1 months' duration that radiates down the right leg. Structural examination reveals the following:

    • positive seated flexion test on the right
    • tenderness and tissue texture change at the right lower pole
    • right ILA resists anterior motion
    • left upper pole is deep

15. The most likely diagnosis is

    A. left anterior sacrum
    B. left posterior sacrum
    C. left unilateral sacral extension
    D. right anterior sacrum
    E. right posterior sacrum

16. Physical examination reveals restriction of internal rotation of the right lower extremity with freedom of external rotation. Which muscle group is most likely involved?

    A. adductors
    B. gluteus maximus
    C. gluteus medius
    D. hamstrings
    E. piriformis

Questions 17-18 refer to the following

A 30-year-old presents with sacroiliac pain. Structural examination reveals a positive seated flexion test on the right, motion restriction at the left lower pole, and a deep right sacral sulcus with associated tissue texture change and tenderness to palpation.

17. The most likely diagnosis is

    A. anterior sacrum left
    B. anterior sacrum right
    C. posterior sacrum left
    D. posterior sacrum right
    E. unilateral sacral extension right

18. Which of the following statements is most associated with sacral counternutation?

    A. during craniosacral flexion the sacral base moves anterior
    B. during craniosacral flexion the sacral base moves posterior
    C. during craniosacral extension the sacral apex moves anterior
    D. during craniosacral extension the sacral base moves anterior
    E. during craniosacral extension the sacral base moves posterior

MATCHING

For each numbered item (description) select one heading (structure) most closely associated with it. Each lettered heading may be selected once, more than once, or not at all.

    A. sacroiliac ligament
    B. sacrospinous ligament
    C. sacrotuberous ligament
    D. tendon of the obturator internus muscle
    E. tendon of the piriformis muscle

19. Divides the greater and lesser sciatic foramen.

    A. A
    B. B
    C. C
    D. D
    E. E

20. Inserts on the ischial tuberosities and becomes taut with terminal flexion.
    A. A
    B. B
    C. C
    D. D
    E. E

Explanations

1. Answer: **A**

    The inferior transverse axis allows for movement of the ilia on the sacrum. It is the hypothetical functional axis of sacral motion that passes from side to side along the anterior convexity of the upper and lower limbs of the sacroiliac joint.

2. Answer: **A**

    This patient has a L-on-L forward sacral torsion. The most important initial findings to review (static findings) are the shallow left ILA and deep right sulcus. The other information confirms the diagnosis. A left-on-left forward torsion will also be associated with springing at the right base – the right superior aspect of the sacrum. There will be resistance to springing of the left ILA due to it being posterior or 'shallow.' There will also be resistance to springing of the poles of the left oblique axis: right ILA and left sulcus. Finally, L5 will exhibit type I Fryette mechanics and be neutral, convex right (sidebent left), rotated right.

3. Answer: **D**

    This patient has a bilateral sacral extension, also known as a posterior sacral base. The dysfunction occurs about the middle transverse axis and is associated with bilateral shallow sacral sulci, deep ILAs, and a positive lumbosacral spring test. The patient has a falsely negative standing/seated flexions test due to both sacroiliac joints being restricted.

4. Answer: **E**

    This patient has a right unilateral sacral flexion, also known as an inferior sacral shear, about a transverse axis. In a sacral shear, the sacral base can appear as if has slipped anteriorly or posteriorly around a transverse axis that allows it to shift within the L-shaped sacroiliac joint. 61 p.595. The base of the sacrum (superior aspect) moves anteriorly during sacral flexion. Structural exam will reveal a deep or anterior right sacral sulcus, inferior and posterior or shallow right ILA, and a positive seated flexion test on the right. Unilateral extensions are associated with superior/anterior ILAs and shallow sacral sulci.

5. Answer: **A**

    This patient has a left anterior innominate rotation, likely due to an ipsilateral quadriceps strain from running. Always refer to the patient's symptoms and standing flexion test when provided information about ASIS/PSIS symmetry to determine the laterality of the dysfunction. In this scenario we are provided information about the right side, however, the left side is affected. For example, if the right ASIS is superior, then the left ASIS is inferior when compared. Other exam findings may include tissue texture changes at the ipsilateral ILA, iliolumbar tenderness, and an ipsilaterally positive ASIS compression test.

6. Answer: **E**

   Of the options provided, the only dysfunction associated with a deep right sacral sulcus is a right unilateral sacral flexion, also known as a sacral shear. These will also have an inferior and posterior right ILA with associated motion restriction and a positive seated flexion test on the right.

7. Answer: **A**

   The patient has a left-on-left sacral torsion which is consistent with a deep right sacral sulcus and a shallow left ILA. The seated flexion test is positive on the opposite side of the sacral axis, in this case positive on the right. The lumbar curve is convex to the right which is the same as sidebent left. L5 exhibits neutral mechanics and will be rotated to the contralateral side of the sacral axis (rotated right) and sidebent to the same side (sidebent left). In a unilateral sacral extension on the right the sacral sulcus will be shallow on the right.

8. Answer: **D**

   A forward sacral torsion on a right oblique axis (right rotation on a right oblique axis) is consistent with the above findings. We know that the left portion of the sacral base (superior portion of the sacrum) has moved anteriorly because of the deep left sacral sulcus and negative lumbosacral spring test. The posterior/inferior ILA on the right this indicates that this portion of the sacrum has moved posteriorly. In a backward sacral torsion or a bilateral sacral extension, the lumbosacral spring test would be positive (i.e. the lumbosacral junction would not spring). In a unilateral sacral flexion on the left, the left ILA would be posterior and significantly inferior.

9. Answer: **D**

   The sacral base is the superior portion of the sacrum and the apex is the inferior aspect. The dysfunction is most likely a forward torsion because of the negative lumbosacral spring test, and the anterior (deep) right sacral base (sulcus) leads us to a diagnosis of a left-on-left sacral torsion. Using the rules of L5 on the sacrum and Fryette's principles one can figure out the dysfunction of L5: 1) When L5 is rotated, the sacrum rotates in the opposite direction. 2) When L5 is sidebent, a sacral oblique axis is engaged on the same side as the sidebending. Fryette's principle I: If L5 is rotated right and sidebent left, L5 must be in the neutral plane. Thus, if the sacrum is rotated left, then L5 must be rotated right. If the sacrum has a left oblique axis, then L5 must be sidebent left. Because L5 sidebends and rotates in opposite directions, then L5 exhibits neutral mechanics. Therefore, L5 is $NS_L R_R$.

10. Answer: **D**

   A right sacral rotation on a right oblique axis will result in a deep sacral sulcus on the left, a posterior/inferior ILA on the right, and the lumbosacral junction springs freely upon compression. A right sacral shear can either be a right unilateral sacral flexion or a right unilateral sacral extension. A right unilateral sacral extension will result in a positive lumbosacral spring test. A right unilateral sacral flexion will result in a deep sacral sulcus on the right (not left).

11. Answer: **C**

   In a sacral torsion (or sacral rotation on an oblique axis) the seated flexion test is positive on the opposite side of the axis. In this case the right positive seated flexion test indicates a left oblique axis. A positive (lumbosacral) spring test indicates that part of the sacral base has moved posteriorly. Since the left sacral base is anterior (i.e., the left sulcus is deep), then this must indicate that the right sacral base has moved posterior. In a right unilateral sacral flexion the right sulcus would be deeper, and the lumbosacral junction would spring freely. In an extended sacral base the seated flexion test would be falsely negative, and the sulci would appear symmetric.

12. Answer: **A**

   The inferior lateral angle (ILA) of the sacrum is the point on the lateral surface of the sacrum where it curves medially to the body of the 5th sacral vertebrae. It is the origin of the sacrotuberous ligament and commonly palpated during the sacral structural examination.

13. Answer: **A**

   Applying anterior pressure on the right ILA will cause the sacrum to rock on a right oblique axis such that the left sacral base (superior aspect of the sacrum) will become shallow or posterior.

14. Answer: **E**

   It is believed that the sacrum moves anteriorly around alternating oblique axes with ambulation as described by Mitchell et al. During swinging of the right lower extremity (left side support), a right pelvic list loads weight on the sacrum creating a left rotation about a left oblique axis (L-on-L). 61 p.585 The other axes are more pertinent for other physiologic motion. Craniosacral and respiratory movements rotate about the superior transverse axis. Postural motion, such as flexion or extension, rotates about the middle transverse axis. Innominates rotate about the inferior transverse axis.

15. Answer: **E**

This patient has a right posterior sacrum which has findings similar to a R-on-L backward sacral torsion. This question may have been challenging because of the reference to the 'poles' in addition to providing a lot of contralateral exam findings. The poles of the oblique axis represent the sacral sulcus in the upper pole and ILA at the lower pole. Structural exam will reveal a shallow right sacral sulcus that restricts compression, an anterior left ILA that springs, positive seated flexion test on the right, and tissue texture changes or tenderness at the right ILA.

16. Answer: **E**

The piriformis muscle externally rotates as well as extends and abducts the thigh with the hip flexed. Because it has attachments to the anterior sacrum, the piriformis can be irritated 63 p.111 when stretched by a posterior sacrum and can therefore contribute to sciatica. Refer to Appendix B to review muscle actions.

17. Answer: **B**

This patient has an anterior right sacrum where the right sacral sulcus has moved anteriorly around an oblique axis. It is similar to a left on left forward sacral torsion. Structural exam will reveal a deep right sacral sulcus, positive seated flexion test on the right, a posterior right ILA (right lower pole), and restriction of springing in the left ILA (left lower pole).

18. Answer: **B**

Counternutation of the sacrum involves posterior motion of the sacral base (superior aspect) which is the same as bilateral sacral extension. This can be confusing because this all occurs during craniosacral flexion, relating to flexion of the cranium where the head is widened and the AP diameter decreases.

19. Answer: **B**

The bilateral sacrospinous ligaments lie anterior to the sacrotuberous ligaments and attach to the ischial spines, diving this space into the greater and lesser sciatic foramen.

20. Answer: **C**

The bilateral sacrotuberous ligaments run from the inferior medial border of the sacrum and insert on the ischial tuberosities and the posterior margins of the sciatic notches.

UPPER EXTREMITIES

Shoulder

I. Anatomy

A. Bones
– Clavicle - acts as a strut for upper limb to allow maximum freedom of motion, as well as transmit forces from the upper extremity to the axial skeleton. It is the only bone connecting the upper extremity and the axial spine.
– Scapula
– Humerus

B. Joints
–Scapulothoracic (pseudo-joint)
–Acromioclavicular
–Sternoclavicular
–Glenohumeral

C. Muscles

1. Rotator cuff - the group of 4 muscles that serve to protect the shoulder joint and give it stability by holding the head of the humerus in the glenoid fossa.[9]
p.537

   mnemonic: **SITS**

   S = supraspinatus - abduction of the arm.
   I = infraspinatus - external rotation of arm.
   T = teres minor - external rotation of arm.
   S = subscapularis - internal rotation of arm.

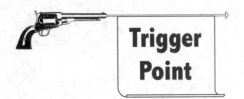

Trigger Point

Know the rotator cuff muscles.

2. Other muscles of the shoulder
   Table 7.1 [1 p.643]

Action	Muscle
Primary flexors	Deltoid (anterior portion), coracobrachialis
Primary extensors	Latissimus dorsi, teres major and deltoid (posterior portion)
Primary abductors	Deltoid (middle portion), supraspinatus
Primary adductors	Pectoralis major, latissimus dorsi
Primary external rotators	Infraspinatus, teres minor
Primary internal rotators	Subscapularis, pectoralis major, latissumus dorsi

D. Arterial supply

– The subclavian artery passes between the anterior and middle scalenes. The subclavian vein passes anterior to the anterior scalene. Therefore, contracture of the anterior and middle scalenes may compromise arterial supply to the arm, but not affect venous drainage.

– The subclavian artery becomes the axillary artery at the lateral border of the first rib.

– The axillary artery becomes the brachial artery at the inferior border of the teres minor muscle.

– The profunda brachial artery is the first major branch of the brachial artery. It accompanies the radial nerve in its posterior course of the radial groove. [9 p.547]

– The brachial artery divides into the ulnar and radial arteries under the bicipital aponeurosis.

– The radial artery courses the lateral aspect of the forearm supplying blood to the elbow, wrist, dorsal aspect of the hand, and eventually forming most of the deep palmar arterial arch.

– The ulnar artery courses the medial aspect of the forearm supplying blood to the elbow, wrist, dorsal aspect of the hand and eventually forming most of the superficial palmar arterial arch.

E. Lymphatic drainage of the upper extremities

Right upper extremity drains into the right (minor) duct.
Left upper extremity drains into the left (main) duct.
For a more detailed description of the lymphatic system see Chapter 13 "Lymphatics."

<u>Treatment to relieve lymph congestion of the upper extremity</u> [7 p. 604]

1. Open the thoracic inlet.
2. Redome the thoraco–abdominal diaphragm.
3. Perform posterior axillary fold technique.

F. <u>Nerves</u>

1. <u>Sympathethic innervation</u> – arises from the upper throacic cord. Dysfunction in the upper thoracics or ribs may increase sympathetic tone to the upper extremity and produce altered motion, nerve dysfunction and lymphatic or venous congestion.[1 p.645]

2. <u>Brachial plexus</u> – responsible for supplying the nerves to the upper extremity. It is composed of nerves from roots C5-C8 and T1. A thorough neurological examination of the upper extremity demands that every physician have a good understanding of the brachial plexus.

Fig 7.1: *The brachial plexus:*

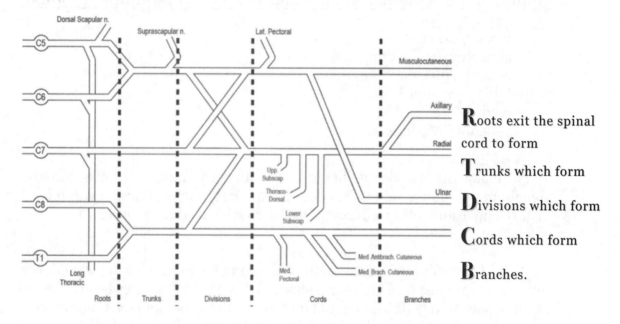

Roots exit the spinal cord to form
Trunks which form
Divisions which form
Cords which form
Branches.

MEMORY TOOL:

Easy way to remember Roots, Trunks, Divisions, Cords, Branches =
Really **T**hirsty? **D**rink **C**old **B**eer!

3. Peripheral nerves –
    a. Median nerve – common sites for entrapment cause:
        Pronator syndrome – entrapment as the median nerve passes through the pronator muscle or at the ligament of Struthers
        Anterior interosseus syndrome
        Carpal tunnel syndrome – described later in this chapter

    b. Ulnar nerve – common sites for entrapment cause
        Cubital tunnel syndrome – entrapment at the elbow
        Entrapment at Guyon's canal (wrist)

    c. Radial Nerve –
        Saturday night palsy – described later in this chapter
        Posterior interosseus syndrome

II. Motion and somatic dysfunction of the upper arm

A. Motion of the shoulder (glenohumeral and scapulothoracic joints)
Glenohumeral joint –
- flexion/extension
- abduction/adduction
- external/internal rotation

Scapulothoracic joint -
- medial/lateral glide
- superior/inferior glide

Normally, the arm can abduct to 180° with active motion, 120° is due to glenohumeral motion and 60° is due to scapulothoracic motion. A careful history and examination will reveal to the physician which joint has a restriction.

A good screening examination for gross range of motion of the shoulder is Apley's Scratch test (see Chapter 18 Special Tests). The Spencer techniques can more accurately test individual motions of the shoulder (see Chapter 17 Articulatory Techniques). This modality can be expanded to include treatment as well.

B. Somatic dysfunction of the shoulder
– Dysfunction of the shoulder joint are active or passive exaggerations of its cardinal movement (flexion/extension, etc)[1 p.652]

C. Motion at the clavicle[1 p. 653, 7 p.163]
– Each end of the clavicle can glide:
– Anterior / Posterior   **OR**   Superior / Inferior

– Motions at either end of the clavicle are in opposite directions.
  – For example, if the lateral end of the clavicle has moved superiorly (e.g. shoulder shrug) the medial end would move inferiorly.
  – Example #2: if the lateral end of the clavicle has moved posterior, the medial end would move anterior.
– The clavicle can also rotate around a transverse axis.
  With flexion of the shoulder (or external rotation with the arm at 90 degrees), the clavicle will rotate posteriorly. With extension of the shoulder (or internal rotation with the arm a 90 degrees) the clavicle will rotate anteriorli).[1 p.653]

1. Sternoclavicular joint
   – Primary somatic dysfunction = Clavicle, anterior and superior on the sternum.[1 p. 653, 7 p. 596]

2. Acromioclavicular joint
   – Primary somatic dysfunction = rotation of the clavicle (around a long axis) is restricted.[1 p.562]
     Anterior rotated clavicle dysfunction is associated with restriction of humeral flexion
     Posterior rotated clavicle dysfunction is associated with restriction of humeral extension.

III. Common problems of the shoulder

A. Thoracic outlet syndrome
Pathogenesis: Compression of the neurovascular bundle (subclavian artery and vein, and the brachial plexus) as it exits the thoracic outlet.
Compression can occur in three places:[7 p.528-9, 1 p.658]
  1. Between the anterior and middle scalenes
  2. Between the clavicle and the first rib
  3. Between pectoralis minor and the upper ribs

Compression may be due to:
  1. A cervical rib
  2. Excessive tension of the anterior or middle scalenes
  3. Somatic dysfunction of the clavicle or upper ribs
  4. Abnormal insertion of pectoralis minor

Location of pain: Shoulder and arm pain
Quality of pain: Ache, paresthesias, weakness, Raynaud phenomenon
Signs and Symptoms: On examination, the scalenes, a cervical rib, or the clavicle may be tender. Pulses in the upper extremity may be normal or diminished. *Often there is a positive Adson's test (if compression between scalenes), Military posture test (if compression between clavicle*

and rib 1) or Hyperextension test (if compression occurs between under pectoralis minor) (see Chapter 18 Special Tests). Sympathetic dysfunction has accompanying palpatory findings in the upper thoraicics and ribs.

Treatment: OMT should be directed at cervical, upper thoracic and rib regions, clavicle, and scalenes if somatic dysfunction is present.[1 p.658,7 p. 528] Exercises to strengthen trapezius and levator scapula.[12 p.463]

B. Rotator cuff tendonitis

Pathogenesis: Inflammation of the tendons of the rotator cuff can be caused by repetitive overuse, trauma, instability of the glenohumeral joint or musculotendinous failure. This most often occurs with the supraspinatus as a result of impingment of the greater tuberosity of the humerus against the acromion.[1 p.658]

Signs and symptoms: The pain is usually exacerbated by abduction, especially from 60°-120°. This is commonly referred to as the "painful arc".

Osteopathic findings:

Cervical somatic dysfunction - can impair nerve function to rotator cuff

Upper thoracic and rib dysfunction - contrubutes to abnormal rotator cuff firing patterns

Lumbar and SI joint dysfunction - can affect the shoulder through latissisumus dorsi tension

Classifications: Neer [46] classified impingment and rotator cuff disease into in three stages:

1) Inflammation and edema
2) Fibrosis and tendonitis
3) Partial or complete tearing

Treatment: Rest, ice and NSAIDS for the acute stages. OMT needs to address the axial component improve scapular mobilty and decrease fascial tension. Physical therapy is critial, but more effective once somatic dysfunction is improved and inflammation diminished.[1 p.658]

C. Bicipital tendonitis

Pathogenesis: An inflammation of the tendon and its sheath of the long head of the biceps. It is usually due to overuse, combined with physiological wear and tear, leading to adhesions that bind the tendon to the bicipital groove. It also may result from a subluxation of the bicepital tendon out of the bicipital groove.[8 p.559]

Location of pain: Anterior portion of the shoulder which may radiate to the biceps.

Signs and symptoms: Tenderness is usually present over the bicipital groove. Pain is usually aggravated by resisted flexion or supination of the forearm.[22 p. 1366]

Treatment: Rest and ice for acute injury. For severe cases, an injection with lidocaine or steriods may provide relief. OMT should include freeing up any restrictions in the glenohumeral area, and myofascial release.

D. Rotator cuff tear

Definition: A tear at the insertion of one of the rotator cuff tendons, usually the supraspinatus. Minor tears of the cuff are common. However, a complete tear can occur resulting in retraction of the affected muscle, and sharp shoulder pain.

Etiology: Often associated with trauma, however can occur as a result of chronic tendonitis

Location of pain: Tenderness just below the tip of the acromion

Quality of pain: A transient sharp pain in the shoulder followed by a steady ache that may last for days [12 p.470]

Signs and symptoms: In supraspinatus tears, a weakness in active abduction is often present along with a *positive drop arm test* (see Chapter 18 Special Tests). Atrophy is a common sign. Often the patient will experience pain for months especially at night.

Treatment: For minor tears, rest, ice and NSAIDS in the acute stages. OMT should be directed at freeing up any restrictions in the glenohumeral area as well as treating the clavicle, upper thoracic, and ribs for somatic dysfunction. Surgery is often required for complete avulsion.

E. Adhesive capsulitis/Frozen shoulder syndrome

Definition: A common condition characterized by pain and restriction of shoulder motion.

Signs and symptoms: Decreased range of motion, with active and passive movements. Abduction, internal and external range of motion is often effected. Extension is typically preserved. Pain is often present at the end of the range of motion.[17 p.98]

Epidemiology: It is most often seen in patients over 40 years of age.[12 p.469]

Etiology: *It is typically caused by prolonged immobility of the shoulder but can occur idiopathically.*

Location of pain: Tenderness is usually at the anterior portion of the shoulder.

Treatment: Early mobilization following shoulder injury is essential. Injection of corticosteriods and NSAIDS may help. OMT includes Spencer techniques, treatment to upper thoracic and ribs.[1 p.658]

F. Shoulder dislocation

Common in athletes and usually occurs as a result of trauma. *Humeral dislocation usually occurs anteriorly.* Recurrent shoulder dislocations are common and require less force. Injury to the axillary nerve can occur with anterior shoulder dislocation.

G. Winging of the scapula

Usually a weakness of the anterior serratus muscle due to a long thoracic nerve injury. This condition is evident if the scapula protrudes posterio-medially while the patient is pushing on a wall.

H. Brachial plexus injuries

The nerves of the brachial plexus are susceptible to traction injury especially during childbirth. *Erb-Duchenne's palsy is by far the most common form of brachial plexus injury. It is an upper arm paralysis caused by injury to C5 and C6 nerve roots usually during childbirth.* It can result in paralysis of the deltoid, external rotators, biceps, brachioradialis, and supinator muscles. Klumpke's palsy is much less common, and is due to injury to C8 and T1. Paralysis usually occurs in the intrinsic muscles of the hand.

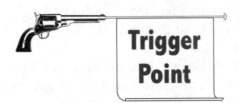

Trigger Point

Most common type of brachial plexus injury is Erb-Duchenne's palsy.

I. Radial nerve injury

The radial nerve is the most common nerve injured in the upper extremity due to direct trauma. It may be injured in the axilla by direct pressure, such as crutch palsy, caused by improper use of **crutches**. More commonly, it is injured as it travels within the spinal groove in **humeral fractures**. **Saturday night palsy** is caused by compression of the nerve against the humerus, as the arm is draped over the back of a chair during intoxication or deep sleep. These injuries typically will result in wrist drop, and possibly triceps weakness depending on the location of the nerve injury.

Elbow, Wrist and Hand

I. Anatomy

A. Bones
- Radius
- Ulna
- Eight carpal bones
- Five metacarpals
- Fourteen phalanges

MEMORY TOOL:

Scaphoid	**S**ome
Lunate	**L**overs
Triquetral	**T**ry
Pisiform	**P**ositions
Trapezium	**T**hat
Trapezoid	**T**hey
Capate	**C**an't
Hamate	**H**andle

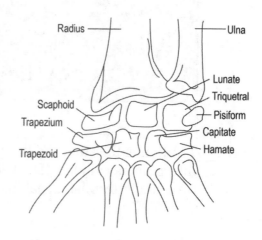

Fig 7.2: The carpal bones

B. Joints
- Elbow (ulna and humerus)
- Ulna and Radius (distal and proximal)
- Intercarpals, carpometacarpals, metacarpophalangeal (MCP), interphalangeal (PIP & DIP).

C Muscles and innervations [1p.644]
- Primary **flexors of the wrist and hand** originate on or near the medial epicondyle of the humerus. Most of which are *innervated by the median nerve* (except for flexor carpi ulnaris – ulnar nerve).
- Primary **extensors** of the wrist and hand originate at the lateral epicondyle of the humerus. *All extensors are innervated by the radial nerve.*
- Primary **supinators** of the forearm are the biceps (*musculocutaneous nerve*) and the supinator (*radial nerve*).
- Primary **pronators** of the forearm are the pronator teres and pronator quadratus (*median nerve*).

D. Muscles of the hand
Muscles in the thenar eminence are innervated by the *median nerve* (except for adductor pollicis brevis which is innervated by the *ulnar nerve*).

Muscles in the hypothenar eminence and interossi are innervated by the *ulnar nerve*.

Lumbricals (4)

First and Second lumbricals are innervated by the *median nerve*.

Third and Fourth lumbricals are innervated by the *ulnar nerve*.

> # MEMORY TOOL:
>
> The **D**eep finger flexors (Flexor digitorum profundus) attach to the **DIP's**

NOTE: Remember that the flexor digitorum profundus attaches to the distal interphalengeal joint (DIP). The flexor digitorum superficialis attaches to the proximal interphalangeal joint (PIP).

II. Motion of the Elbow and Forearm

A. **Carrying angle** (Fig. 7.3)
-Formed by the intersection of two lines. The first line is the longitudinal axis of the humerus. The second line starts at the distal radial-ulna joint, and passes through the proximal radial ulna joint.
-The normal carrying angle in men is 5°.
-The normal carrying angle in women is 10°-12°.
-A carrying angle > 15° is called cubitus valgus, or abduction of the ulna if somatic dysfunction is present.
-A carrying angle < 3° is called cubitis varus or, adduction of the ulna if somatic dysfunction is present.

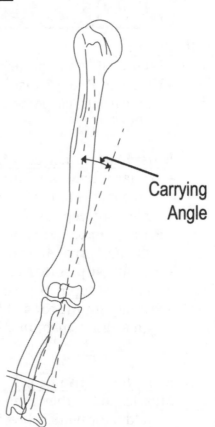

Fig. 7.3: The angle formed between the two dotted lines represents the carrying angle.

B. Carrying angle and its inflluence on the wrist

Due to a parallelogram effect, **an increase in the carrying angle (abduction of the ulna) will cause an adduction of the wrist.**

Conversely, **a decrease in the carrying angle (adduction of the ulna) will cause an abduction of the wrist.**[1p.651]

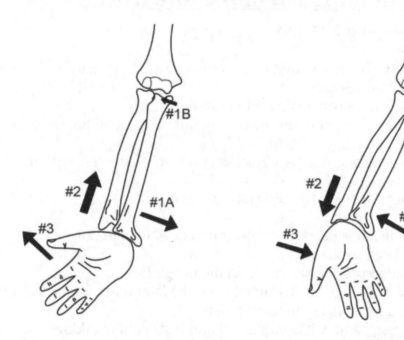

Fig. 7.4: *Adduction of the ulna (arrow #1A) and lateral glide of the olecranon (proximal ulna) (arrow #1B) will cause the radius to be pulled proximally (arrow #2). This will result in abduction of the wrist (arrow #3).*

Fig. 7.5: *Abduction of the ulna (arrow #1A) and medial glide of the olecranon (proximal ulna) (arrow #1B) will cause the radius to be pushed distally (arrow #2). This will result in adduction of the wrist (arrow #3).*

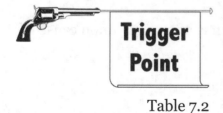

Table 7.2

Carrying Angle	Ulna Movement	Wrist Movement
Increased	Abduction	Adduction
Decreased	Adduction	Abduction

C. **Radial head motion**
   The radial head will glide anteriorly and posteriorly with supination and
   pronation respectively of the forearm.[1p.655]
   When the forearm is pronated, the radial head will glide posteriorly.
   When the forearm is supinated, the radial head will glide anteriorly.

III. Somatic dysfunction of the forearm

A. **Abduction of the ulna** (See figure 7.5)
   Findings:[1p.655, 10p.239]
   -Carrying angle increased (olecranon deviated medially and distal ulna
      deviated laterally).
   -Olecranon process restricted in lateral glide.
   -Radial head may be compressed against the lateral humeral condyle
   -Distal ulna resticted in medial glide.
   -The wrist/hand will be adducted and restricted in abduction.

B. **Adduction of the ulna** (See figure 7.4)
   Findings:[1p.655, 10 p.240]
   -Carrying angle decreased (olecranon deviated laterally and distal ulna
      deviated medially).
   -Olecranon process restricted in medial glide.
   -Radial head may be distracted from the lateral humeral condyle.
   -Distal ulna resticted in lateral glide.
   -The wrist/hand will be abducted and restricted in adduction.

C. **Posterior radial head**
   Etiology:
   -Falling forward on a pronated forearm is often a common cause.[1p.655]
   Findings:[10p.242]
   -Restricted supination of the forearm.
   -Restricted anterior glide of the radial head.

D. **Anterior radial head**
   Etiology:
   Falling backward on a supinated forearm is often a common cause.[1p.655]
   Findings:[10p.244]
   -Restricted pronation of the forearm.
   -Restricted posterior glide of the radial head.

E. **Interosseous membrane dysfunction** - the interosseous membrane can
   retain stress patterns of past injury therefore this can perpetuate elbow or
   wrist disability even after proper orthopedic care.[1p.654] Palpation of the
   interosseous membrane will reveal increased tension and tenderness. This
   can be treated with direct or indirect myofascial release.

IV. Motion and Somatic dysfunction of the wrist

A. Wrist motion

With **wrist flexion**, *the three proximal carpal bones that articulate with the radius will glide* **dorsally.**

With **wrist extension**, *the three proximal carpal bones that articulate with the radius will glide* **ventrally.**

B. Somatic Dysfunction

1) Wrist extension somatic dysfunction
   - Wrist restricted in flexion.
   - Carpal bones glide ventrally and are restricted in dorsal glide

2) Wrist flexion somatic dysfunction
   - Wrist restriced in extension.
   - Carpal bones glide dorsally and are restricted in ventral glide
   - ***Most common wrist somatic dysfunction***[1p.656]

V. Common complaints of the wrist and elbow

A. Carpal tunnel syndrome

Definition: Entrapment of the median nerve at the wrist.[17 p.192]

Quality and location of pain: *The patient usually complains of paresthesias of the thumb and the first 2 ½ digits.*

Signs and symptoms: Weakness and atrophy usually appear late. On examination, symptoms are reproduced with Tinel, Phalen, and prayer tests.

Diagnosis: Nerve conduction studies/electromyography remain the gold standard.

Treatment: Treatment usually consists of splints, NSAIDS, and steroid injections. Surgery is indicated if medical treatment has failed.

Osteopathic treatment for carpal tunnel syndrome:[1 p.657]

1. Treating rib and upper thoracic somatic dysfunctions to decrease sympathetic tone in the upper extremity.
2. Treating cervical somatic dysfunctions and myofascial restrictions to enhance brachial plexus function and remove potential sites of additional compression.
3. Direct release techniques to increase the space in the carpal tunnel.

B. Lateral epicondylitis (tennis elbow)

Definition: A strain of the extensor muscles of the forearm near the lateral epicondyle.

Pathogenesis: Commonly develops as a result of overuse of the forearm extensors and supinators. Aggravating activities include hitting a ball in racquet sports with improper techniques, and turning a screwdriver.[17 p.139]

Location of pain: The patient usually complains of pain over the lateral epicondyle that worsens with wrist extension against resistance.[61 p.658]

Quality of pain: Pain may radiate to the lateral aspect of the arm and forearm.

Signs and symptoms: Tenderness will be present at the lateral epicondyle or just distal to it. Pain often worsens with activity.

Treatment: NSAIDS, rest, and ice. To prevent reoccurrences, a tennis elbow strap worn just below the elbow often helps.[17 p.141] OMT should be directed toward correcting cervical or upper thoracic dysfunctions, counterstrain to affected muscles (usually extensors), and myofascial release to decrease fascial restrictions.

C. **Medial epicondylitis (golfer's elbow)**

Definition: A strain of the flexor muscles of the forearm near the medial epicondyle.

Pathogenesis: Commonly develops as a result of overuse of the forearm flexors and pronators.[17 p.139]

Location/quality of pain, signs/symptoms, treatment: Same for tennis elbow but directed at the medial epicondyle.

VI. <u>Deformities of the hand</u>

A. **Swan-neck deformity** (Fig. 7.6)
- -Flexion contracture of the MCP and DIP.
- -Extension contracture of the PIP.
- -Results from a contracture of the intrinsic muscles of the hand and is often associated with rheumatoid arthritis.

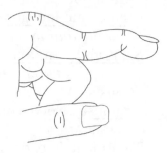

Fig 7.6: *Swan neck deformity*

B. **Boutonniere deformity** (Fig. 7.7)
- -Extension contracture of the MCP and DIP.
- -Flexion contracture of the PIP.
- -Results from a rupture of the hood of the extensor tendon at the PIP and is often associated with rheumatoid arthritis.

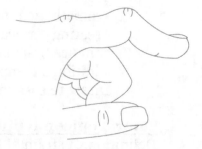

Fig 7.7: *Boutonniere deformity*

Review Questions

1. A middle-aged male had a sudden syncopal event and a good samaritan comes to the man's aid. The first responder palpates the patient's pulse on the distal portion of the lateral wrist. Which one of the following statements is associated with the most likely vessel that is being palpated for pulse?

    A. It branches directly from the profunda brachial artery and accompanies the radial nerve in the posterior course of the radial groove
    B. It branches directly from the axillary artery supply the lateral aspect of the forearm
    C. It branches directly from the axillary artery supply the medial aspect of the forearm
    D. forms most of the deep palmar arch of the hand
    E. forms the first major branch of the brachial artery

2. A surgeon is releasing restrictions in the upper extremity of a man suffering from thoracic outlet syndrome and locates the brachial artery. The origin of this structure is at the

    A. inferior border of teres minor
    B. inferior/lateral border of the clavicle
    C. lateral border of the first rib
    D. superior border of pectoralis minor
    E. superior border of teres minor

3. An 18-year-old presents with acute shoulder pain and an obvious bony deformity. Plain film radiography reveals a dislocated humerus. Which of the following is the most likely location of this patient's shoulder dislocation?

    A. anterior
    B. inferior
    C. inferior and posterior
    D. lateral
    E. posterior

4. A 21-year-old presents to your office with right shoulder pain of several weeks' duration. History reveals he is a right-handed pitcher for a minor league baseball team. Physical examination reveals tenderness at the tip of the acromion and a positive drop arm test. Range of motion testing reveals pain with abduction, especially between 60 and 120 degrees. The most likely diagnosis is

   A. a cervical rib
   B. adhesive capsulitis
   C. bicipital tenosynovitis
   D. rupture of the supraspinatus tendon
   E. supraspinatus tendonitis

5. A 30-year-old presents with forearm pain. Physical examination reveals increased forearm pain with resisted wrist extension. Palpatory tenderness is likely expected over the

   A. bicipital aponeurosis
   B. humeral condyles
   C. lateral epicondyle
   D. medial epicondyle
   E. olecranon

6. An 23-year-old presents with wrist drop. Physical examination reveals mild sensory loss to the dorsum of the hand. The most likely structure injured is the

   A. dorsal branch of the ulnar nerve
   B. median nerve
   C. musculocutaneous nerve
   D. palmar interosseous nerve
   E. radial nerve

7. A child presents with forearm pain after playing tag on the playground. Structural examination reveals an abducted ulna somatic dysfunction. The most likely associated structural exam finding is

   A. abduction of the wrist
   B. cubitus varus
   C. decreased carrying angle
   D. medial glide of the olecranon
   E. proximal radial glide

8. A 30-year-old presents with upper back pain of 3 months duration. Physical examination reveals a prominent medial border of the scapula with arm flexion during a push-up motion against a wall. The most likely injured nerve is:

   A. axillary
   B. long thoracic
   C. lower subscapular
   D. suprascapular
   E. spinal accessory

Questions 9-10 refer to the following:

A 31-year-old female presents to your office with neck pain following a motor vehicle accident two days ago. She describes a dull ache on the right side of her neck that radiates into her arm. Physical examination reveals a tenderpoint of the right anterior scalene and a diminished radial pulse with inspiration during ipsilateral shoulder extension, abduction and external. Neurological exam reveals that sensation is intact, there is 5/5 muscle strength, and normal deep tendon reflexes.

9. The most likely diagnosis is

    A. bicipital tenosynovitis
    B. herniated nucleus pulposus of the cervical spine
    C. thoracic outlet syndrome
    D. rotator cuff tear
    E. supraspinatus tendonitis

10. Compression has most likely occurred between the

    A. anterior scalene and clavicle
    B. cervical rib and the upper ribs
    C. joint of Luschka and facet joint
    D. middle and posterior scalene muscles
    E. pectoralis minor and the upper ribs

Questions 11-12 refer to the following:

A young adult presents for a pre-participation sports physical without complaints. Vitals and physical examination are unremarkable.

11. The examiner palpates the carpal bones. Which of the following is the most medial structure?

    A. capitate
    B. hamate
    C. scaphoid
    D. trapezoid
    E. trapezium

12. The examiner then assesses pronation and supination of the forearm. Pronators of the forearm are primarily innervated by which one of the following nerves?

    A. deep branch of the radial nerve
    B. dorsal branch of the ulnar nerve
    C. median nerve
    D. musculocutaneous nerve
    E. superficial branch of the radial nerve

Questions 13-15 refer to the following:

A 12-year-old presents with chronic upper extremity paresis due to a known injury to the C5 and C6 nerve roots during childbirth.

13. The most likely diagnosis is

    A. Bell's palsy
    B. Erb-Duchenne palsy
    C. Klumpke's palsy
    D. long thoracic nerve palsy
    E. stick palsy

14. The most likely associated finding upon neurologic examination is

    A. decreased biceps reflex
    B. decreased sensation over the medial epicondyle
    C. decreased sensation over the ring and little finger
    D. increased triceps reflex
    E. weak finger flexors

15. Which of the following nerves primarily carries fibers from the C5 nerve root?

    A. dorsal scapular
    B. lateral pectoral
    C. long thoracic
    D. musculocutaneous
    E. thoracodorsal

Questions 16-17 refer to the following:
A 35-year-old female presents with numbness and tingling over the palmar surface of her right thumb of 6 months duration that is worse at night. History reveals it often radiates into her first and middle fingers. Physical examination reveals a decreased sensation at the pads of the first and middle fingers with a decreased grip strength of the right hand.

16. The most likely diagnosis is

    A. de Quervain tenosynovitis
    B. carpal tunnel syndrome
    C. cubital tunnel syndrome
    D. radial sensory nerve entrapment
    E. scaphoid fracture

17. Which of the following structures is most likely contributing to symptoms?

    A. abductor pollicis longus tendon
    B. median nerve
    C. scapholunate ligament
    D. superficial radial nerve
    E. ulnar nerve

Questions 18-19 refer to the following:

A 15-year-old female presents with left wrist and elbow pain of 1 weeks' duration. Physical examination reveals tenderpoints at the elbow and wrist. Structural examination reveals a decreased carrying angle and a wrist that restricts adduction. Radiography is negative for acute boney abnormalities.

18. The most likely diagnosis is

    A. abducted ulna
    B. adducted ulna
    C. anterior radial head
    D. interosseous membrane dysfunction
    E. posterior radial head

19. Osteopathic manipulation is performed and the ulna somatic dysfunction resolves. The examiner reassesses the extremity with focus on the radial head. He gently moves the arm to cause the radial head to glide anteriorly. Which of the following movements will facilitate this motion?

    A. extension of the elbow
    B. extension of the wrist
    C. flexion of the wrist
    D. pronation of the forearm
    E. supination of the forearm

MATCHING

For each numbered item (description) select one heading (associated muscle) most closely associated with it. Each lettered heading may be selected once, more than once, or not at all.

    A. infraspinatus
    B. subscapularis
    C. supraspinatus
    D. teres major
    E. teres minor

20. Primary abductor of the humerus.

    A. A
    B. B
    C. C
    D. D
    E. E

21. A female presents with shoulder pain after playing tug-of-war. An MRI is obtained and reveals the rotator cuff muscles to be unremarkable.

    A. A
    B. B
    C. C
    D. D
    E. E

Explanations

1. Answer: **D**

The bystander is palpating the patient's radial artery which is a division of the brachial artery that courses on the lateral aspect of the forearm. It eventually forms the deep palmar arterial arch. The profunda brachial artery is the first major branch of the brachial artery which accompanies the radial nerve in the radial groove and supplies the lateral elbow (answer A). Branches from the brachial artery (not axillary – answers B and C) supply the medial and lateral forearm via the radial and ulnar arteries. The first major branch of the brachial artery is the profunda brachial artery (answer E).

2. Answer: **A**

The axillary artery is a continuation of the subclavian artery at the lateral border of the first rib. The brachial artery is the continuation of the axillary artery beyond the inferior border of the teres minor muscle. It is palpable in the antecubital fossa medial to the bicipital tendon and divides into the radial and ulnar arteries.

3. Answer: **A**

Anterior dislocations are the most common (95%), posterior dislocations are the second (2-4%), and inferior dislocations are the least common (0.5%).

4. Answer: **E**

The supraspinatus is a primary abductor of the arm and also assists in external rotation. The supraspinatus can also be tested in the 'empty can' position by abducting in the scapular plane (30 degrees flexed forward) with internal rotation. Rupture would have resulted in profound loss of range of motion and likely the inability to continue pitching. Biceps tendinopathy typically results in pain when carrying objects with the elbows bent or lifting overhead; there may be pain with resisted elbow flexion or supination as well as tenderness in the bicipital groove. Adhesive capsulitis results in a significant loss of range of motion in both passive and active phases.

5. Answer: **C**

The lateral epicondyle is the origin for most wrist extensors and can be inflamed with repeated extension and supination. Symptoms include localized tenderness over the lateral epicondyle and pain with resisted wrist extension with the elbow in full extension, or lateral epicondyle pain with passive terminal wrist flexion.

Medial epicondylitis is also known as golfer's elbow due to the inflammation caused by repeated wrist flexion and pronation. The bicipital aponeurosis is a flat, broad tendon of the biceps brachii in the cubital fossa.

6. Answer: **E**

The radial nerve is predisposed to compression in spiral groove of the humerus and may cause wrist drop if compressed. Symptoms include weakness of the wrist and finger extensors as well as the brachioradialis with sensory loss over the dorsal hand, possibly extending up the posterior forearm.

7. Answer: **D**

During abduction of the ulna the distal ulna is deviated laterally away from the body. The olecranon is on the proximal ulna and glides medially, thus resisting lateral glide. The radius glides distally, and the wrist is laterally pushed into increased adduction and would resist abduction. Increased abduction of the ulna would increase the carrying angle causing cubitus valgus (distal forearm away from the midline of the body).

8. Answer: **B**

This patient is exhibiting scapular winging due to damage of the long thoracic nerve, a purely motor nerve that arises from C5-C7 and innervates the serratus anterior. Associated findings include a scapula that is displaced more medially and superiorly. Lateral scapular winging (in which the scapula glides laterally) can be due to damage of the spinal accessory nerve that innervates the trapezius; this form is elicited by arm abduction and external rotation against resistance.

9. Answer: **C**

Thoracic outlet syndrome is a constellation of signs and symptoms due to compression of the upper neurovascular bundle by various structures. The Adson's test is supportive and described here as being positive as supported by a diminished or absent radial pulse (see Chapter 18 Special Tests). Symptoms are dependent upon the structure compressed. Neurologic compression may result in pain, weakness, numbness in the hand, arm, or shoulder. Arterial compression can cause arm or hand ischemia and subsequently pain, paresthesia, pallor, or coolness. Venous compression can lead to swelling, cyanosis, or venous thrombosis.

10. Answer: **E**

Thoracic outlet syndrome most commonly occurs between the scalene triangle (anterior and middle scalenes and first rib), costoclavicular space (first rib and clavicle), or pectoralis minor space (pectoralis minor and upper ribs). A cervical rib will compress the scalene triangle. While the other options are theoretically plausible, neither is as common as the three spaces described above. Note that the joint of Luschka is formed between uncinate processes and the uncus of the cervical vertebrae and is a common cause of nerve root compression (radiculopathy), not a cause of thoracic outlet syndrome.

11. Answer: **B**

The hamate is the most medial bone of the group provided, forming a hook-like process into the palmar surface. Recall the mnemonic: Some Lovers Try Positions That They Can't Handle, which names the carpal bones lateral to medial in first the proximal, then distal rows. The order is as follows: (proximally) scaphoid, lunate, triquetral, pisiform; (distally) trapezium, trapezoid, capitate, hamate.

12. Answer: **C**

The median nerve innervates several muscles involved with pronation as well as all of the flexors of the forearm (except for flexor carpi ulnaris and a portion of the flexor digitorum profundus which are supplied by the muscular branches of the ulnar nerve). Specific pronators innervated include the pronator teres and pronator quadratus. Compression of the median nerve as it passes through the pronator teres muscle may cause pronator syndrome. This can cause pain in the proximal volar forearm and sensory symptoms in the radial 3 1/2 digits and is aggravated by elbow flexion against resistance.

13. Answer: **B**

Erb's palsy or Erb-Duchenne palsy results in paralysis of the arm due to injury of the C5-C6 nerve roots (occasionally C7). This causes the arm to be held in adduction, internal rotation, and forearm extension due to weakness of the deltoid and infraspinatus muscles (mainly C5) and biceps (mainly C6). Klumpke's palsy is less common and due to injury of C8-T1, resulting in isolated hand paralysis. Paralysis of the long thoracic nerve will result in scapular winging. Bell's palsy is a transient weakness of facial muscles. Some use 'stick palsy' as an alternate term for a trigger finger.

14. Answer: **A**

The C5-C6 nerve root correlates to the biceps and brachioradialis deep tendon reflexes and provides sensation to the lateral elbow and lateral forearm/thumb, respectively. The motor action of C5 is primarily elbow flexion while the motor action of C6 is wrist extension. The triceps reflex correlates to the C7-C8 nerve roots. Refer to Appendix B to review the peripheral nerve distribution in the upper extremity.

15. Answer: **A**

The dorsal scapular nerve arises directly from the C5 nerve root with occasional innervation from C4.[9p.522t] The dorsal scapular nerve innervates the rhomboid and levator scapulae muscles. The lateral pectoral nerve arises from C5, C6, and C7 nerve roots. The long thoracic nerve from C5, C6, and C7 nerve roots. The musculocutaneous nerve from C5 and C6 nerve roots. The thoracodorsal nerve from C6,C7, and C8 nerve roots [9p.522t]

16. Answer: **B**

Carpal tunnel syndrome is due to compression of the median nerve as it travels through the carpal tunnel. This may cause pain or paresthesia to the thumb and the first 2 and 1/2 digits. Symptoms are usually worse at night or exacerbated by activities involving flexion or extension of the wrist. Clinical signs may include weakness of thumb abduction and opposition as well as atrophy of the thenar eminence. Sensory loss is a early finding involving the median-innervated fingers, weakness and atrophy appear late. A positive Phalen sign is defined as reproduction of symptoms after 1 minute of wrist flexion. A positive Tinel's sign is defined as a reproduction of symptoms with percussion over the median nerve at the carpal tunnel. See the explanation below regarding the distractor options.

17. Answer: **B**

See the explanation above regarding carpal tunnel syndrome. De Quervain tendinopathy affects the abductor pollicis longus and extensor pollicis brevis tendons and is associated with pain on the radial side of the wrist. Ulnar or cubital tunnel syndrome results in weakness of the dorsal interosseous muscles thus decreasing grip strength, however it is associated with 4th and 5th digit paresthesia. Radial sensory nerve entrapment causes paresthesias over the dorsum of the hand, wrist, and first three digits. Scaphoid fractures can occur after a fall onto an outstretched hand and are associated with pain or swelling in the anatomic snuffbox with possible separation of the scapholunate ligament. This patient has no traumatic history to lead us to consider a scaphoid fracture.

18. Answer: **B**

During adduction of the ulna the distal ulna is deviated medially toward the body. Increased adduction of the ulna would decrease the carrying angle causing cubitus varus (distal forearm toward the midline of body). This would encourage abduction of the hand at the wrist, which would resist adduction. Interosseous membrane dysfunction can result in tension and tenderness of the interosseous tissues long after an injury and must be treated with direct or indirect fascial treatments.

19. Answer: **E**

Supination of the forearm will cause the radial head to glide anterior. Pronation will cause the radial head to glide posterior. Anterior radial head dysfunctions are typically caused by a fall backward (supinated position), while posterior radial head dysfunctions are caused by a fall forward onto an outstretched hand (pronated position) because these respective movements cause anterior/posterior motion of the radial head.

20. Answer: **C**

The supraspinatus and deltoid (midportion) are primary abductors of the glenohumeral joint.[1p.643] The supraspinatus is supplied by the suprascapular nerve. The serratus anterior via scapula and deltoid (anterior, posterior) muscle are secondary abductors.

21. Answer: **D**

This item is essentially asking you to choose the muscle that is NOT part of the rotator cuff. The teres major is a medial rotator and adductor of the humerus. It works with the latissimus dorsi muscle to cause humeral extension, internal rotation, and adduction. All of the other distractors are part of the rotator cuff; recall the mnemonic SITS.

Lower Extremities 8

Hip and Knee

I. Anatomy

A. Bones and bony landmarks

1. <u>Femur</u> - proximally articulates with the acetabulum; distally articulates with the medial and lateral menisci that are situated on the tibial plateau.
2. <u>Patella</u> - a sesamoid bone that attaches to the quadriceps tendon superiorly, and the patella tendon inferiorly.
3. <u>Tibia</u>
4. <u>Fibula</u>

B. Muscle of the hip and knee

1. <u>Hip</u>
   Primary extensor: Gluteus maximus
   Primary flexor: Iliopsoas

2. <u>Knee</u>
   Primary extensor: Quadriceps (rectus femoris, vastus lateralis, medialis and intermedius)
   Primary flexors: Semimembranosus and semitendinosus (hamstrings)

C. Ligaments and joints

1. Hip

   a. Femoroacetabular joint (hip joint) - a ball and socket joint that is held in place by the surrounding musculature and four ligaments.
      1) Iliofemoral ligament - also known as the "Y- ligament of Bigelow." This is the strongest ligament in the body.
      2) Ischiofemoral ligament
      3) Pubofemoral ligament
      4) Capitis femoris - the ligament at the head of the femur attaching to the acetabular fossa.

   b. Hip motion and somatic dysfunction
      1) Major motions
         - Flexion/Extension
         - Abduction/Adduction
         - Internal rotation/External rotation
      2) Minor motions
         - Anterior glide
           The head of the femur will glide anteriorly with external rotation of the hip.[1 p.606]
         - Posterior glide
           The head of the femur will glide posteriorly with internal rotation of the hip.[1 p.606]
      3) Somatic dysfunction of the hip (table 8.1)

External rotation somatic dysfunction	Internal rotation somatic dysfunction

Findings:
   Hip restricted in internal rotation
	Findings:
	   Hip restricted in external rotation

Etiology:
   Piriformis or iliopsoas spasm
	Etiology:
	   Spasm of internal rotators (gluteus. minimus, semimembranosus, semitendinosus., TFL, adductor. magnus, adductor. longus.)

2. Knee
   The knee is composed of three joints and four major ligaments.

   a. Tibiofemoral joint - the largest joint in the body [23 p.372] The articular surfaces of the tibia and femur are separated by two "C" shaped menisci.[23 p.372] The medial and lateral menisci act as shock absorbers and also aid in nutrition and lubrication of the joint. Between the two menisci are two ligaments that help stabilize the knee:
      1) The anterior cruciate ligament (ACL) - originates at the posterior aspect of the femur, and attaches to the anterior aspect of the tibia. *It prevents anterior translation of the tibia on the femur.*

2) <u>The posterior cruciate ligament (PCL)</u> - originates on the anterior aspect of the femur and inserts on the posterior aspect of the tibia. *It prevents posterior translation of the tibia on the femur.*

3) <u>Medial collateral ligament (tibial collateral ligament)</u> - originates at the femur and inserts on the tibia. This ligament also articulates with the medial meniscus.

4) <u>Lateral collateral ligament (fibular collateral ligament)</u> - originates at the femur and inserts on the fibula.

c. <u>Patellofemoral joint</u> - Posterior aspect of the patella as it tracks in between the medial and lateral femoral condyles

d. <u>Tibiofibular joint</u> - a synovial joint composed of the lateral aspect of the proximal tibia and the proximal fibular head. Movement at this joint can occur with pronation and supination of the foot or internal and external rotation of the tibia. [1] p.612

- *The fibular head will glide anteriorly with external rotation of the tibia.*
  External rotation of the tibia and ankle will push the distal fibula posteriorly; reciprocally, the proximal fibular will move anteriorly.

- *The fibular head will glide posteriorly with internal rotation of the tibia.*
  Internal rotation of the tibia and ankle will pull the distal fibula anteriorly; reciprocally, the proximal fibula will move posteriorly.

- *The fibular head will glide anteriorly with pronation of the foot.* (Fig. 8.1)
  Pronation (dorsiflexion, eversion and abduction) of the foot causes ligamentous structures to push the distal fibula posteriorly; reciprocally, the proximal fibular will move anteriorly. [1] p.612

- *The fibular head will glide posteriorly with supination of the foot.* (Fig. 8.2)
  Supination (plantarflexion, inversion and adduction) of the foot causes ligamentous structures to pull the distal fibula anteriorly; reciprocally, the proximal fibular will move posterior. [61] p.612

Fibular head movement:

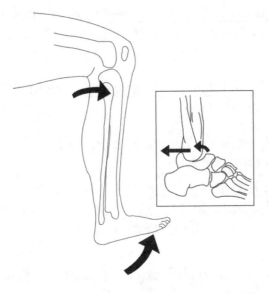

Fig 8.1: *Fibular head movement. Pronation at the foot will cause the fibular head to glide anteriorly.*

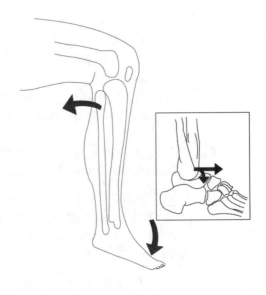

Fig 8.2: *Supination at the foot will cause the fibular head to glide posteriorly.*

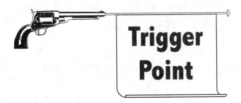

Trigger Point

1. **Dorsiflexion, eversion, and abduction = PRONATION of the foot.**
2. **Plantarflexion, inversion, and adduction = SUPINATION of the foot.**

I. Nerves

A Femoral nerve - (L2-L4)
Motor - innervates quadriceps, iliacus, sartorius and pectineus.
Sensory - anterior thigh and medial leg.

B. Sciatic nerve - (L4-S3) Courses through the greater sciatic foramen. In 85% of the population the sciatic nerve will be inferior to the piriformis muscle.
Two divisions:

1. Tibial
   a. Motor - Hamstrings except short head of the biceps femoris, most plantar flexors, and toe flexors.
   b. Sensory - Lower leg and plantar aspect of foot.

2. Peroneal
   a. Motor - Short head of biceps femoris, evertors and dorsiflexors of the foot, and most extensors of the toes.
   b. Sensory - Lower leg and dorsum of foot.

III. Anatomical variations of the femur and Q angle (quadriceps angle)

A. Angulation of the head of the femur (Figs. 8.3 a-c)
The normal angle between the neck and shaft of the femur is 120° -135°.
*If this angle is < 120° this condition is called **coxa vara**.*[1 p.606]
*If this angle is > 135° this condition is called **coxa valga**.*[1 p.606]

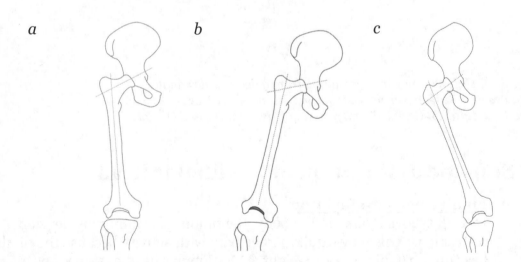

Fig. 8.3a (left): *Normal angle between the neck and shaft of the femur is approximately 120°-135°.*
Fig. 8.3b (middle): *Coxa valga; the angle between the neck and the shaft of the femur is >135°.*
Fig. 8.3c (right): *Coxa vara; the angle between the neck and the shaft of the femur is <120°.*

B. <u>Q angle</u> (Figs. 8.4a-c)

The Q angle is formed by the intersection of a line from the ASIS through the middle of the patella, and a line from the tibial tubercle through the middle of the patella. A normal Q angle is 10° - 12°.[1] p.610 *An increased Q angle is referred to as genu valgum*, in which the patient will appear more knocked-kneed. *A decreased Q angle is referred to as genu varum*, in which the patient will appear more bowlegged.[1] p.610

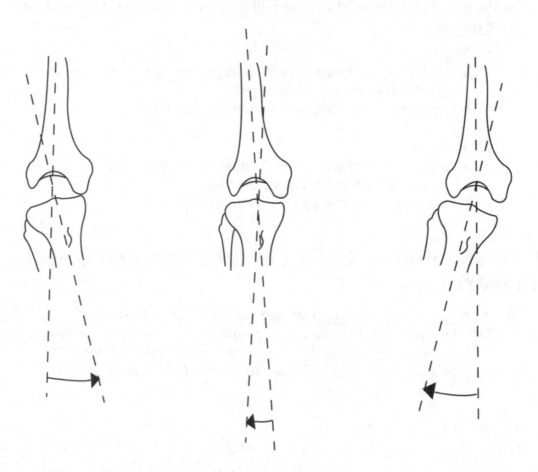

Fig. 8.4a (left): *Genu varum, resulting from a decreased Q angle.*
Fig. 8.4b (middle): *Normal Q angle approximately 10°-12°.*
Fig. 8.4c (right): *Genu valgum, resulting from an increased Q angle*

IV. Somatic dysfunction of the fibular head

A. <u>Fibular head dysfunction</u>

Like all synovial joints in the body, the tibiofibular joint may develop restrictions. This may result in knee pain with activity because the fibula can bear up to 1/6 of the body weight.[23] p. 374 Fibular head dysfunctions often occur in recurrent ankle sprains. In the more common supination sprain, the proximal fibular will be posterior.[1] p.612

Two somatic dysfunctions are possible with fibular head movement: (table 8.2)

Posterior fibular head	Anterior fibular head
Findings:[10 p.292] - Proximal fibular head resists anterior spring. - Distal fibula may be anterior and resists posterior springing. - Talus is internally rotated which causes foot to invert and plantarflex.	Findings:[10 p.295] - Proximal fibular head resists posterior spring. - Distal fibula may be posterior and resists anterior springing. - Talus externally rotated causing foot to evert and dorsiflex.

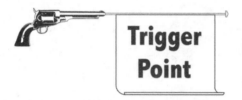

Trigger Point

The common peroneal nerve (common fibular nerve) lies directly posterior to the proximal fibular head. Therefore, a posterior fibular head or fracture of the fibula may disturb the function of this nerve.

V. Clinical considerations of the hip and knee

A. Patello-femoral syndrome

Pathophysiology: An imbalance of the musculature of the quadriceps (strong vastus lateralis and weak vastus medialis). This imbalance will cause the patella to deviate laterally, and eventually lead to irregular or accelerated wearing on the posterior surface of the patella. The quadriceps imbalance is generally thought to be due to biomechanics related to a larger Q angle [1 p.610]

Signs and Symptoms: Deep knee pain is present, especially when climbing stairs. The physician may notice atrophy in the vastus medialis, and often the patient will have patella crepitus.

Prevalence - Mostly in women. A wider pelvis often results in a larger Q angle.

Treatment - Strengthen the vastus medialis muscle.

B. Ligamentous sprain classification
Three grades of sprains. [1 p.605]
    a. <u>First degree</u>: no tear resulting in good tensile strength and no laxity
    b. <u>Second degree</u>: partial tear resulting in a decreased tensile strength with mild to moderate laxity
    c. <u>Third degree</u>: complete tear resulting in no tensile strength and severe laxity

<u>NOTE</u>: In most cases, third degree sprains may require surgery, while first and second degree sprains generally can be treated conservatively.

C. Compartment syndrome
Usually results from trauma or vigorous overuse leading to an increase in intracompartmental pressure. This will compromise circulation within that compartment.

The lower leg can be divided into four compartments:
1. Anterior
2. Lateral
3. Deep posterior
4. Superficial posterior

The anterior compartment is most often affected.[17 p.9] This often results in severe unrelenting pain after and during exercise. The anterior tibilais muscle is hard and tender to palpation, pulses are present and stretching the muscle causes extreme pain.[17 p.10] Treatment usually consists of ice and myofascial release, to increase venous and lymph return. Since muscle necrosis can develop within 4 to 8 hours, if intracompartmental remains elevated a surgical fasciotomy is indicated.[8 p.655]

D. O'Donaghue's triad

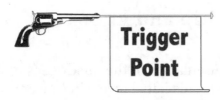
Trigger Point

O'Donaghue's triad (terrible triad): a common knee injury resulting in the injury to the ACL, MCL and medial meniscus.

Ankle and foot

I. Anatomy

This region consists of 26 bones, 55 articulations, 30 synovial joints, and supported by over 100 ligaments and 30 muscles.

A. Bones (Fig. 8.5)
Talus
Calcaneus
Navicular
Cuboid
3 Cuneiforms
5 Metatarsals
14 Phalanges

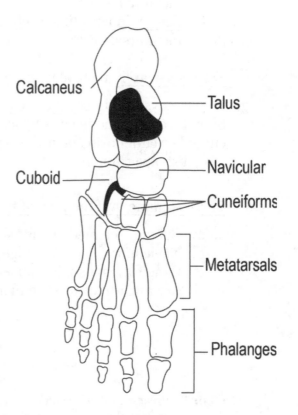

Fig. 8.5: Bones of the foot: Note the gray area of the talus, (trochlea of the talus). This portion of the talus articulates with the ankle mortise. It is wider anteriorly, making the foot more stable in dorsiflexion.

B. Joints

1. Talocrural joint (tibiotalar joint): a hinge joint located between the talus and the medial malleolus of the tibia, and the lateral malleolus of the fibula.[23 p.448]

   Main motions = plantar flexion and dorsiflexion
   Minor motions = anterior glide of the talus (with plantar flexion) and posterior glide of the talus (with dorsiflexion).
   Due to the configuration of the talus and the ankle mortise, the ankle is more stable in dorsiflexion than plantar flexion (see Fig. 8.5). This is the reason why 80% of ankle sprains occur in plantar flexion.[1 p.614]

2. Subtalar joint (talocalcaneal joint): acts mostly as a shock absorber, and also allows internal and external rotation of the leg while the foot is fixed.

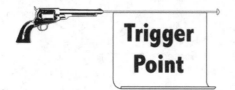
Trigger Point

The ankle is more stable in dorsiflexion.

C. Arches

1. Longitudinal arches:
   a. Medial longitudinal arch: talus, navicular, cuneiforms, 1st to 3rd metatarsals.[1 p.618]
   b. Lateral longitudinal arch: calcaneus, cuboid, and 4th and 5th metatarsals.[1 p.618]

2. Transverse arch: navicular, cuneiforms, and cuboid

3. Somatic dysfunction of the arches
   Somatic dysfunctions usually occur within the transverse arch. The navicular, cuboid or cuneiforms be may displaced, causing pain. This is often seen in long distance runners.

   Three somatic dysfunctions of the transverse arch: (fig 8.6) [1 p.619]

   a. Cuboid: the medial edge will glide toward the plantar surface.
   b. Navicular: the lateral edge will glide toward the plantar surface.
   c. Cuneiforms: usually caused by the second cuneiform gliding directly downward, toward the plantar surface.

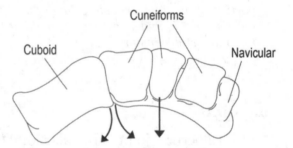

Fig 8.6: Transverse arch of the foot. It is composed of the cuboid, cuneiforms, and the navicular. Arrows show three possible somatic dysfunctions

D. Ligaments

Since there are over one hundred ligaments in the foot and ankle, we are going to limit our discussion to the major stabilizing ligaments.

1. Lateral stabilizers of the ankle: These ligaments prevent excessive supination.

   a. Anterior talofibular ligament
   b. Calcaneofibular ligament
   c. Posterior talofibular ligament

   Fig 8.7: Lateral stabilizers of the ankle

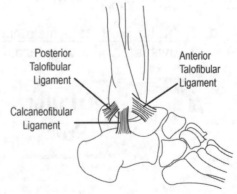

<u>Important note</u>: Due to the less stable supination position of the ankle, sprains often cause damage to these ligaments. *The most common injured ligament is the anterior talofibular ligament.*[25] *Sprains associated with the supination position are classified into 3 types depending on the extent of ligamentous injury.*[1 p.615]

<u>Type I</u>: involves the anterior talofibular ligament.
<u>Type II</u>: involves the anterior talofibular ligament and the calcaneofibular ligament.
<u>Type III</u>: involves the anterior talofibular ligament, calcaneofibular ligament and the posterior talofibular ligament.

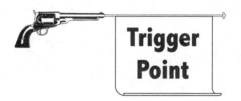

Trigger Point

The most common injured ligament in the foot is the Anterior Talofibular ligament (ATF) =Always Tears First.

2. <u>Medial stabilizer of the ankle</u>: This ligament prevents excessive pronation.
    a. <u>Deltoid ligament</u>: Since the ankle is more stable in the pronation position and the deltoid ligament is very strong, pronation sprains are very uncommon. Excessive pronation usually results in a fracture of the medial malleolus rather than pure ligamentous injury.

3. <u>Plantar ligaments</u>
    a. <u>Spring ligament (calcaneonavicular ligament)</u>: This ligament strengthens and supports the medial longitudinal arch.
    b. <u>Plantar aponeurosis (plantar fascia)</u>: Strong, dense, connective tissue that originates at the calcaneus and attaches to the phalanges. Chronic irritation to this structure may cause calcium to be laid down along the lines of stress, leading to a heel spur.[8 p.639]

Chapter 8 Review Questions

1. A 65-year-old female presents with right low back and hip pain after gardening yesterday. Structural examination reveals hypertonicity and pain with passive motion testing of the primary flexor of the hip. The most likely muscle involved is the

   A. gluteus medius
   B. gluteus maximus
   C. hamstrings
   D. iliopsoas
   E. quadriceps

2. A pro football player is hit by another player and develops acute knee pain. Physical examination reveals excessive anterior translation of the tibia . The most likely structure injured is the

   A. anterior cruciate ligament
   B. posterior cruciate ligament
   C. lateral collateral ligament
   D. medial collateral ligament
   E. patellar complex

3. An 18-year-old soccer player sustains an injury to multiple structures referred to as the "the terrible triad" or "O'Donaghue's triad." Which of the following were most likely injured?

   A. anterior cruciate ligament, medial meniscus, and lateral collateral ligament
   B. anterior cruciate ligament, medial meniscus, and lateral meniscus
   C. anterior cruciate ligament, medial meniscus, and medial collateral ligament
   D. anterior cruciate ligament, lateral meniscus, and lateral collateral ligament
   E. posterior cruciate ligament, medial meniscus, and lateral collateral ligament

4. A high school football player presents with leg pain after a long practice. Structural examination reveals the fibular head resists anterior glide. Which of the following is most associated with this dysfunction?

   A. it often occurs following a supination ankle sprain
   B. plantarflexion of the ankle will be restricted on the affected side
   C. the distal fibular head may be posterior
   D. the proximal fibula will resist posterior glide
   E. the talus will be externally rotated on the affected side

5. A 3-year-old presents for a well child examination and the parents are concerned about the way the child walks. Roentgenoograhic examination reveals a decrease in the angle between the neck and the shaft of the femur. The most likely diagnosis is

    A. a decreased Q angle
    B. coxa valga
    C. coxa vara
    D. genu valgum
    E. genu varum

6. A 4-year-old presents for a well child examination and the parents are concerned about the appearance of the child's legs. Physical examination reveals a decreased Q angle. Which of the following is most associated with this abnormal finding?

    A. bow-legged appearance
    B. coxa vara
    C. genu valgum
    D. knock-knees appearance
    E. patellofemoral syndrome

7. A female nursing home patient rolls her ankle on a curb and develops acute pain and swelling. Examination reveals the associated ligament to likely have at least a portion of the fibers disrupted. The most likely diagnosis is a

    A. first degree sprain
    B. second degree sprain
    C. third degree sprain
    D. fourth degree sprain
    E. fifth degree sprain

8. A tennis player sustains an inversion injury to the anterior talo-fubular and calcaneo-fibular ligaments. Which of the following somatic dysfunctions is most associated with this type of injury?

    A. abducted tibia
    B. adducted medial malleolus
    C. anterior fibular head
    D. anterior lateral malleolus
    E. posterior lateral malleolus

9. An anatomist is researching the stability of the ankle mortise. The ankle is most stable in which one of the following positions?

    A. dorsiflexion
    B. eversion
    C. inversion
    D. plantarflexion
    E. supination

10. A track runner trips and sustains a type II supination ankle sprain. Which of the following structures is most likely injured?

    A. anterior talofibular ligament
    B. anterior talofibular and calcaneofibular ligaments
    C. anterior talofibular, calcaneofibular, and posterior talofibular ligaments
    D. calcaneofibular and posterior talofibular ligaments
    E. deltoid ligament

11. A little league player is struck in the lateral knee with a bat and is subsequently having difficulty ambulating. Plain film radiography reveals a fracture of the fibular head. This type of injury will most likely to affect the

    A. common peroneal nerve
    B. femoral nerve
    C. sciatic nerve
    D. sural nerve
    E. tibial nerve

12. A middle-aged male presents with knee discomfort on the medial side. Structural examination reveals an ipsilateral posterior innominate rotation. The most likely muscle responsible for his knee pain is the

    A. biceps femoris
    B. quadriceps
    C. sartorius
    D. semimembranosus itendinosus
    E. tensor fascia latae

13. A patient presents concerned about the appearance of her flat feet. Structural examination of the lateral longitudinal arch is unremarkable. The most likely bone involved is the

    A. 4th metatarsal
    B. 5th metatarsal
    C. calcaneus
    D. cuboid
    E. navicular

Questions 14-15 refer to the following:
    A middle-aged female presents for consultation of chronic anterior knee pain. History reveals her primary care physician diagnosed her with impaired lateral femoral patella tracking.

14. Which of the following additional features will most likely be discovered upon obtaining further history and examination?

    A. Crepitation of the posterior patella
    B. deep knee pain that worsens at rest
    C. hemorrhagic knee effusion
    D. male gender
    E. positive Lachman's test

15. Treatment involves focused strengthening of the

   A. gastrocnemius
   B. hamstrings
   C. rectus femoris
   D. vastus lateralis
   E. vastus medialis

MATCHING

For each numbered item (description) select one heading (ankle ligament) most closely associated with it. Each lettered heading may be selected once, more than once, or not at all.

   A. anterior talofibular
   B. calcaneofibular
   C. calcaneonavicular
   D. deltoid
   E. posterior talofibular

16. Has tibio-navicular fibers

   A. A
   B. B
   C. C
   D. D
   E. E

17. Most often injured in supination ankle sprains

   A. A
   B. B
   C. C
   D. D
   E. E

Explanations

1. Answer: **D**

   The iliopsoas is a primary flexor of the hip. It originates from the anterior portions of the upper lumbar vertebrae and joins the iliacus to insert on the lesser trochanter of the femur. The gluteus maximus is a primary extensor of the hip. The semimembranosus and semitendinosus (hamstrings) are the primary flexors of the knee while the rectus femoris and vastus lateralis/medialis/oblique (quadriceps) are the primary extensors of the knee.

2. Answer: **A**

   The ACL is an important stabilizing ligament whose primary function is to control anterior translation of the tibia. Its secondary function is to restrain tibial rotation as well as varus and valgus stress. As the knee is extended the tibia translates anteriorly, tightening the ACL and preventing hyperextension. The ACL is comprised of two bundles: an anteromedial bundle that is tight in flexion and a posterolateral bundle that is tight in extension.

3. Answer: **C**

   O'Donaghue's triad involves the ACL, MCL, and medial meniscus. The medial meniscus is typically involved due to its anatomical attachment to the MCL. Note however that recent studies have supported a higher incidence of lateral meniscal involvement with acute injuries in athletes rather than the medial meniscus. [26]

4. Answer: **A**

   This patient has a posterior fibular head dysfunction where the fibular head (proximal fibula) will be posterior and the distal fibula will be anterior. The fibular head will glide posteriorly with supination of the foot and internal rotation of the tibia. Foot supination involves plantarflexion, inversion, and adduction and causes the anterior talofibular ligament to pull the distal fibula anteriorly. A supination ankle sprain can contribute to a posterior fibular head. Findings may also include restriction of dorsiflexion, resistance of anterior glide of the fibular head, and a talus that restricts posterior glide.

5. Answer: **C**

Coxa vara is a deformity of the hip where the angle between the head and the shaft of the femur is <120 degrees resulting in a short leg. It usually presents by age 2 with an abnormal gait. Coxa valga is the opposite of this when the angle is >135 degrees and may result in a long leg. The latter is caused by a slipped epiphysis of the femoral head.

6. Answer: **A**

The Q angle is formed from the intersection of a line drawn from the ASIS through the center of the patella and a line drawn from the center of the patella and the tibial tubercle. The angle is typically smaller in men than compared to women. Genu varum is referred to as having a bow-legged appearance with an angular deformity at the knee with the distal leg toward the midline. The differential for children includes normal physiologic development, Blount disease, rickets, and a multitude of other metabolic and skeletal abnormalities. Genu valgum or knock-knees is the opposite of this.

7. Answer: **B**

The classification for degree of ligamentous sprain includes the following: First degree is either no tear or only microscopic tears with minimal to no laxity. Second degree is a partial tear with mild to moderate laxity, and a third degree is a complete tear with significant instability. There is no such thing as a fourth or fifth degree sprain.

8. Answer: **D**

Injury to the anterior talo-fibular and calcaneo-fibular ligaments implies a supination/inversion injury. This injury will result in the anterior movement of the distal fibular head, hence an anterior lateral malleolus dysfunction. This dysfunction is very similar to a posterior fibular head dysfunction. If the distal fibula moves anteriorly (with ankle inversion) then the proximal fibula moves posteriorly. Fibular movement in this fashion is associated with ankle inversion, the distal fibula glides anteriorly with supination of the foot. Supination involves inversion, plantarflexion, and adduction.

9. Answer: **A**

Dorsiflexion is most stable since this is the position that has the most bone contact on the ankle mortise. The talus is wider anteriorly and narrower posteriorly. (see Fig. 8.5) With dorsiflexion the wider portion of the tibia sits in the ankle mortise, while with plantarflexion the shallow portion of the talus sits in the mortise. The latter allows for more lateral movement, but at the expense of stability.

10. Answer: **B**

Supination involves inversion, plantarflexion, and adduction. A type I supination sprain only involves the anterior talofibular (ATF) ligament while a type II also includes the calcaneofibular ligament. A type III additionally includes the posterior talofibular ligament. The medial deltoid ligament complex is the strongest of the ankle ligaments, but forceful eversion can cause a sprain. Note that the ankle sprain 'types' are a different paradigm than ankle sprain 'degrees,' which relate to the degree of ligamentous damage and instability involved.

11. Answer: **A**

The common peroneal nerve is also known as the common fibular nerve. It is a division of the sciatic nerve and is prone to compression as it wraps around the lateral aspect of the proximal fibula before dividing into deep and superficial branches. Compression or injury results in foot drop with weakened dorsiflexion and a steppage gait.

12. Answer: **C**

The sartorius originates at the ASIS and inserts on the anteromedial surface of the upper tibia in the pes anserinus. The pes anserinus refers to conjoined tendons of the gracilis, sartorious and semitendinosus. It works to flex, abduct, and externally rotate the hip. Those with posterior innominate rotations may develop a secondary sartorius dysfunction due to lengthening of the muscle. [1 p.588]

13. Answer: **E**

The longitudinal arch is supported by the tibialis posterior muscle and divided into medial and lateral components. [1 p.618] Pes planus results in a loss of the medial longitudinal arch. The medial longitudinal arch consists of the talus, navicular, three cuneiforms, and first three metatarsals. The lateral longitudinal arch consists of the calcaneus, cuboid, and 4th and 5th metatarsals.

14. Answer: **A**

Lateral femoral patella tracking is a type of patellofemoral syndrome where the patella is displaced laterally with knee movements. It is associated with accelerated wear on the posterior surface of the patella (chondromalacia patella). [1 p.611] It is more common in women due to a larger Q angle and causes deep knee pain worse when climbing stairs or repetitive knee flexion/extension. [1 p.154] Recurrent dislocation of the patella associated with improper tracking can result from myofascial tension in the quadriceps. If the condition is unilateral, tibial internal rotation, external rotation, or glide dysfunction on the femur should be considered. Hemorrhagic knee effusions are associated with ACL tears.

15. Answer: **E**

Weakness of the vastus medialis (and specifically the vastus medialis obliquus fibers) and hip adductors can contribute to lateral subluxation of the patella. A possible cause is muscle asymmetry with weak medial vs. strong lateral vastus musculature causing the patella to deviate laterally. Over time this leads to accelerated wear on the posterior patella and altered patellar tracking.

16. Answer: **D**

The deltoid ligament is a strong ligament that attaches the medial malleolus to the tarsus. [5 p.488] It consists of four parts, tibionavicular, anterior and posterior tibiotalar and tibiocalcanean. The deltoid ligament complex is the strongest of the ankle ligaments. The deltoid ligament is so strong that it often results in an avulsion fracture of the medial malleolus.

17. Answer: **A**

Supination of the foot involves plantarflexion, inversion, and adduction. This motion will result in a lateral ankle sprain and may involve the anterior talofibular (ATF), calcaneofibular, and posterior talofibular ligaments. The ATF is usually the first or only ligament injured in the vast majority of lateral ankle sprains. Recall the mnemonic "ATF = Always Tears First."

Osteopathy in the Cranial Field

9

I. Introduction

The cranial field was established by William Garner Sutherland D.O., D.Sc (Hon) (1873-1954). Sutherland, who graduated from the American School of Osteopathy, was an early student of A.T. Still. As a student, Sutherland noticed that the articular surfaces of the cranial bones had a unique design. After years of research and careful observations he noticed that the central nervous system (CNS), cerebral spinal fluid (CSF), dural membranes, cranial bones and sacrum functioned as a unit. He named this unit the primary respiratory mechanism (PRM). [1 p.729]

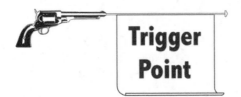

Trigger Point

CNS + CSF + Dural Membranes + cranial bones + sacrum = PRM [1 p.729]

The CNS, CSF, dural membranes, cranial bones and sacrum (PRM) function together as a physiological unit to control and regulate pulmonary respiration (which Sutherland termed *secondary respiration*), circulation, digestion, and elimination.

The PRM is composed of five anatomical-physiological elements. [1 p.730]

1. The inherent rhythmic motion of the brain and spinal cord.
2. Fluctuation of cerebrospinal fluid.
3. Mobilityof intracranial and intraspinal membranes.
4. Articular mobility of cranial bones.
5. Involuntary mobility of sacrum between ilia.

A. The inherent rhythmic motion of the brain and spinal Cord

The brain and spinal cord have a subtle inherent slow pulse-wavelike motion. [1,p.730] The brain and spinal cord lengthens and thins during the exhalation phase and shortens and thickens during the inhalation phase of the primary respiratory mechanism. [27] Several studies outlined in the <u>Foundation of Osteopathic Medicine</u> [1,p.731] have agreed to the pulsatile or piston-like effect of the brain and spinal cord.

B. Fluctuation of the cerebrospinal fluid

CSF movement in a fluctuant flow pattern through the ventricles of the brain and within the subarachnoid space is a well-established phenomenon.

C. Mobility of intracranial and intraspinal membranes

The intracranial and intraspinal membranes (i.e. meninges), surround, support, and partition the CNS. The meninges have three membranes:

1. Dura mater
   The dura mater is the outermost membrane. It is thick, inelastic and forms the *falx cerebri and tentorium cerebelli. The dura projects caudally down the spinal canal, with firm attachments at foramen magnum and S2.* There are occasional attachments at C2, C3 and the lower lumbar region. [1,p.730]
2. Arachnoid mater
3. Pia mater

The intracranial and intraspinal membranes surround support and partition the CNS. The rhythmic motion of the brain and spinal cord, and the fluctuation of the cerebrospinal fluid will cause these membranes to move. Since the dura is inelastic and is attached to the cranial bones, any motion of the dura will influence the cranial bones. Therefore, the meninges will act as an inelastic rope causing the cranial bones to move in response to the rhythmic motion of the brain and spinal cord, and fluctuation of the cerebrospinal fluid. Sutherland called this "inelastic rope" the **Reciprocal Tension Membrane (RTM)**. The RTM has been referred to as the *core link* because of the potential to transmit biomechanical forces linking the cranium to the sacrum.

D. Articular mobility of the cranial bones

Sutherland discovered rhythmic impulses could be palpated on a human skull. Later this was called the **"Cranial Rhythmic Impulse"** or the CRI.[27,p.24] The C.R.I. is commonly reported to be 10 - 14 cycles per minute in most major osteopathic texts.[1 p.735, 27 p.25, 28 p.165, 29 p.140, 30 p.122]

E. Involuntary mobility of the sacrum between the ilia

The inherent motility of the brain and spinal cord, and the fluctuation of CSF will cause the RTM to move. Since a portion of the RTM (the dura) *attaches to the posterior superior aspect of the second sacral segment,* any motion of the RTM will cause the sacrum to move. Research has shown that a slight rocking motion of the sacrum occurs about a *transverse axis that runs though the superior transverse axis of the sacrum located near S2 just posterior to the spinal canal.* [1 p.735]

II. Physiologic motion of the primary respiratory mechanism

The sphenobasilar synchondrosis (SBS) is the articulation of the sphenoid with the occiput. It is the keystone of all cranial movement. The SBS is moved through a biphasic cycle (*flexion and extension*), in response to the pull of the dural membranes. This is influenced by the coiling and uncoiling of the CNS, and the fluctuation of the CSF. [8 p.904]

A. There are two motions that can occur at the SBS:

1. Flexion

– *During flexion, the midline bones of the cranium (sphenoid, occiput, ethmoid, vomer) move through a flexion phase. The paired bones of the cranium will move through an external rotation phase.* An easy way to remember this relationship is:

During "fl **ex** ion" of midline bones,

external rotation of paired bones occur.

– *Flexion at the SBS will cause the dura to be pulled cephalad, moving the sacral base posteriorly through the superior transverse axis of the sacrum. This movement at the sacral base (originally termed sacral extension) is called* **counternutation** (Fig 9.1).

– *Flexion will widen the head slightly and decrease its anterioposterior diameter* (Fig 9.2).

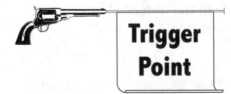

Trigger Point

> ## Craniosacral Flexion:
> 1. **Flexion of the midline bones.**
> 2. **Sacral base posterior (counternutation).**
> 3. **Decreased AP diameter of the cranium.**
> 4. **External rotation of paired bones.**

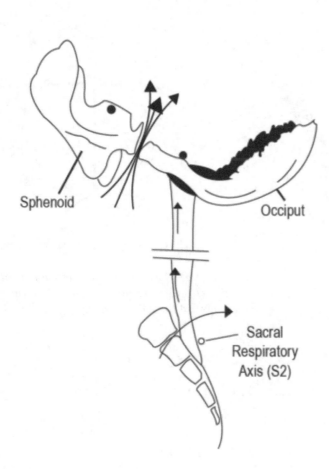

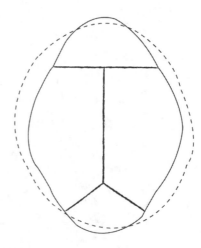

Fig 9.2: Craniosacral flexion (dotted lines) will widen the head slightly and decrease the AP diameter.

Fig 9.1: Flexion of the SBS will cause the dura to be pulled cephalad, resulting in counternutation of the sacrum.

2. **Extension**
    − *During extension, the midline bones of the cranium (sphenoid, occiput, ethmoid, vomer) move through a extension phase. The paired bones of the cranium will move through an internal rotation phase.*
    − *Extension at the SBS will cause the dura to fall caudad, moving the sacral base anterior through the superior transverse axis of the sacrum. This movement at the sacral base (originally termed sacral flexion) is called* **nutation** *(Fig 9.3).*
    − *Extension will narrow the head slightly and increase its anterioposterior diameter (Fig 9.4).*

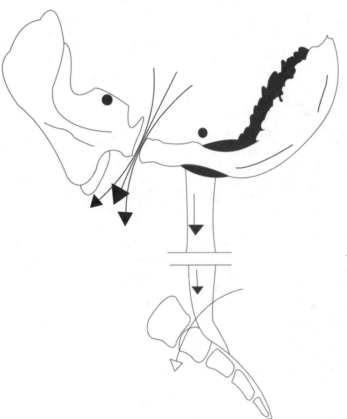

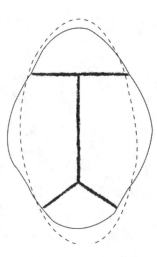

Fig 9.4: *Craniosacral extension (dotted lines) will narrow the head slightly and increase the AP diameter.*

Fig 9.3: *Extension of the SBS will cause the dura to fall caudad, resulting in nutation of the sacrum.*

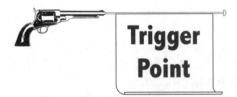

Trigger Point

Craniosacral Extension:
1. **Extension of the midline bones**
2. **Sacral base anterior (nutation)**
3. **Increased AP diameter of the cranium**
4. **Internal rotation of the paired bones**

MEMORY TOOL:

An easy way to distinguish craniosacral flexion from extension is to identify the movement of the sphenoid.

– In craniosacral flexion, the sphenoid looks like it is flexing forward.

– In craniosacral extension, the sphenoid looks like it is extending.

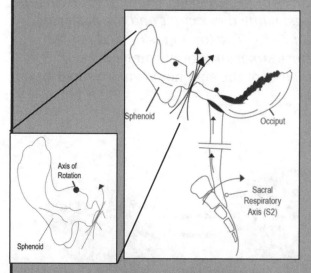

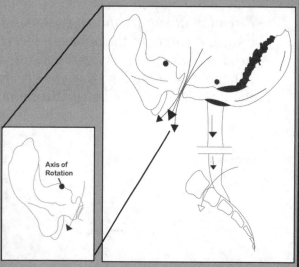

–Therefore one could say that you name craniosacral flexion and extension in the direction of sphenoid movement.

In addition, MOST (not all) craniosacral strains are named for which direction the sphenoid has moved. See specific strains for details.

III. Strains of the sphenobasilar synchondrosis

From before birth until death, the body is subject to strains and stresses. Childbirth, traumatic brain injury, musculoskeletal dysfunction, surgery, and even everyday emotional stress are all examples of strains and stresses that may cause the PRM to be compromised. There are six types of strains that can occur at the SBS. They are:[1 p.737, 27 p.36]

1. Flexion and extension
2. Torsion
3. Sidebending and rotation
4. Vertical strain
5. Lateral strain
6. Compression

A. <u>Torsion</u>

A torsion is a type of strain that occurs when there is a twisting at the SBS. *The sphenoid and other related structures of the anterior cranium rotate in one direction about an anterioposterior axis, while the occiput and the posterior cranium rotate in the opposite direction.*[8 p.906] *The torsion is named for the greater wing of the sphenoid that is more superior.* For example, if the sphenoid is rotated, so that the greater wing of the sphenoid is more superior on the right, this is called a right torsion.

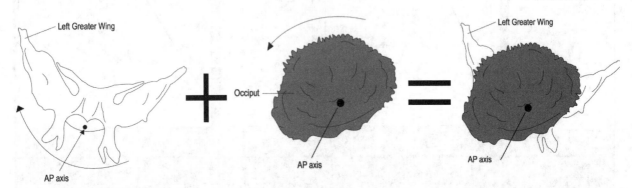

Fig. 9.5a: Posterior view of sphenoid rotating clockwise, such that the left greater wing is superior.

Fig. 9.5b: Posterior view of occiput rotating counter-clockwise.

Fig. 9.5c: Putting together figures a & b produces a left cranial torsion.

B. <u>Sidebending/Rotation</u>

This type of strain has two distinct motions that occur simultaneously about three separate axes. Rotation occurs about an AP axis through the SBS (same axis as a torsion strain) (Fig. 9.6b). However, unlike a torsion, in this type of strain the sphenoid and the occiput rotate in the same direction. Both bones will either rotate clockwise or counterclockwise. Sidebending occurs about two parallel vertical axes - one axis passes through foramen magnum and the other through the center of the sphenoid (Fig. 9.6a). Motion will occur about these two axes so that the SBS will deviate to the right or to the left. Due to the upward convexity of the SBS, sidebending to the left (deviation of the SBS to the left) will cause the sphenoid and occiput to rotate so that they are inferior on the left. This is denoted as SBR$_\text{L}$.

<u>NOTE</u>: the above strains (right torsion, left torsion, SBR$_\text{L}$, SBR$_\text{R}$) are all considered physiologic if their presence does not interfere with the flexion or extension components of the mechanism.[1 p.737]

a

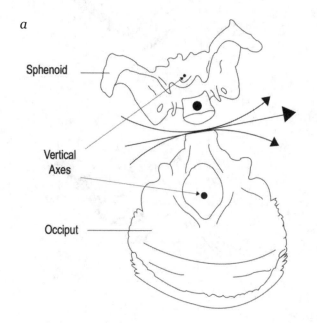

Sphenoid

Vertical
Axes

Occiput

b

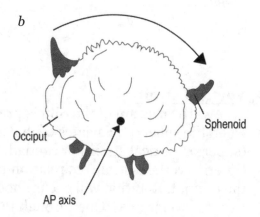

Occiput

Sphenoid

AP axis

Fig. 9.6a: Right sidebending of the SBS about two vertical axes will cause the SBS to deviate to the right.
Fig. 9.6b: Right rotation of the SBS about an AP axis.

C. **Flexion/Extension**

As mentioned earlier, flexion and extension are natural physiologic components of cranial movement. A strain pattern occurs when the mechanism does not move through flexion and extension equally. *An extension lesion occurs when the SBS deviates caudad, decreasing the amount of flexion at the SBS. (Fig 9.7a). Conversely, a flexion lesion occurs when the SBS is deviates cephalad, decreasing the amount of extension at the SBS (Fig 9.7b).*

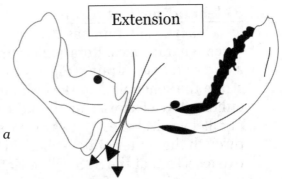

a

Fig. 9.7a: Extension of the SBS. The SBS deviates caudad (arrows) decreasing the amount of flexion at the SBS.

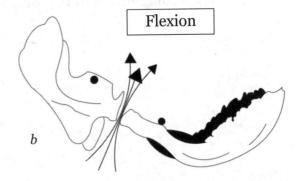

b

Fig. 9.7b (right): Flexion of the SBS:. The SBS deviates cephalad (arrows) decreasing the amount of extension at the SBS.

D. **Vertical strain**

A vertical strain of the SBS is present when the sphenoid deviates cephalad (superior vertical strain) or caudad (inferior vertical strain) in relation to the occiput. Rotation will occur about two transverse axes. One through the center of the sphenoid, the other superior to the occiput (Fig. 9.8)

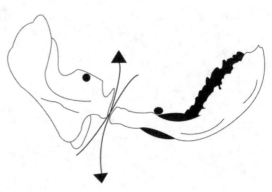

Fig 9.8: Superior vertical strain. The sphenoid deviates cephalad in relation to the occiput.

E. <u>Lateral strain</u>

A lateral strain of the SBS is present when the sphenoid deviates laterally in relation to the occiput. If the sphenoid deviates to the left, it is termed a left lateral strain. If the sphenoid deviates to the right, it is termed a right lateral strain. Rotation will occur about two vertical axes, one through the center of the sphenoid, the other through foramen magnum. Palpation of a lateral strain will feel as if the cranium is shaped like a parallelogram.

<u>NOTE</u>: Vertical and lateral strains may be superimposed on other strains.

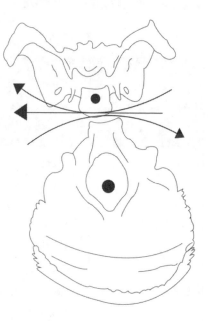

Fig 9.9:   Left lateral strain. The sphenoid deviates laterally in relation to the occiput.

F. <u>Compression</u>

This type of strain occurs when the sphenoid and occiput have been pushed together. As a result there will be a decrease in the amplitude of the flexion and extension components of the CRI. If the compression is severe enough the CRI can be almost completely obliterated.[11 p.135] It can be due to trauma to the back or front of the head or from circumferential compression such as childbirth.[61 p.738]

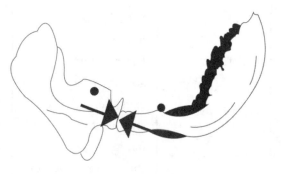

Fig 9.10:   SBS compression

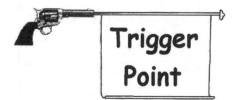

Trigger Point

Compression strain of the SBS can result in severely decreased C.R.I. It can be due to trauma, especially to the back or front of the head or childbirth.[61 p.737]

IV. Cranial nerves

Table 9.1   Summary of the cranial nerves [1. p. 496-497]

Nerve	Exits the cranium	Somatic Dysfunction	Symptoms associated with the Dysfunction
CN I	Cribiform plate		Altered sense of smell
CN II	Optic canal	Sphenoid, occiput	
CN III	Superior orbital fissure	Petrosphenoid ligament	Diplopia, ptosis or accomodation problems
CN IV	Superior orbital fissure		Diplopia
CN V V1	Superior orbital fissure	Temporal	Decreased sensation to the eyelid and scalp
V2	Foramen rotundum		*Trigeminal neuralgia*
V3	Foramen ovale		*Trigeminal neuralgia, headache*
CNVI	Superior orbital fissure		Medial strabismus
CNVII	Enters internal acoustic meatus and exits the stylomastoid foramen.	Sphenoid, temporal, occiput, cervical and thoracic spine	Bell's palsy
		Sphenoid,temporal, occiput	
CNVIII	Int'l acoustic meatus	Temporal, occiput	Tinnitus, vertigo or hearing loss
CN IX	Jugular foramen	Temporal, occiput, OA, AA, C2	
CN X	Jugular foramen		Referred pain and parasymphathetic reflexes
CNXI	Spinal division (C1-C6) enters foramen magnum joins with the cranial division and exits the jugular foramen	Temporal, occiput	Tenderness in the SCM or trapezius
CN XII	Hypoglossal canal	Occiput	Dysphagia

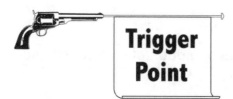

Trigger Point

1. **Vagal somatic dysfunction can be due to OA, AA and/or C2 dysfunction.**[1 p.506, 20 p.58]
2. **Dysfunction of CN VIII can cause tinnitus, vertigo or hearing loss.**
3. **Dysfunction of the condylar portion of the occipital bone (condylar compression (CN XII) can result in poor suckling in the newborn.**
4. **The jugular foramen lies along the occipitomastoid suture (occiput and temporal bones). Occipitomastoid compression can lead to venous congestion and may effect CN IX, X and XI** [1 p.495]

V. Craniosacral treatment

Goals of treatment:[1 p.743]

1. Normalize nerve function (cranial, spinal and autonomic nerves)
2. Normalizing function of cerebrum, thalamus, hypothalamus and pituitary body
3. Normalize arterial, venous and lymphatic channels
4. Normalize CSF fluctuation
5. Release membranous tension
6. Correct cranial articular strains
7. Modify gross structural patterns.

A. Vault hold

Purpose – Assess the PRM and identify the degree of participation of each bone in cranial motion.[32 p.576]

Finger placement for the vault hold is as follows:[32 p.576, 21 p.410]

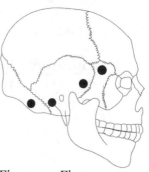

Index finger – greater wing of the sphenoid
Middle finger – temporal bone in front of the ear
Ring finger – mastoid region of temporal bone
Little finger – squamous portion of the occiput

Fig.9.11:   Finger placement for vault hold.

B. <u>Fronto-occipital hold</u>
<u>Purpose</u> – Assess the PRM and identify freedom of motion of the occiput and frontal bones.[32 p.577]

C. <u>Decompression of the occipital condyles</u>
<u>Purpose</u> – Balance the RTM at the hypoglossal canal, normalizing CN XII.[29 p.578]

D. <u>Venous sinus technique</u>
The venous sinuses drain approximately 85 - 95% of the blood from the cranium. The remaining 5% of venous blood drains via the facial veins and external jugular.[29 p.6, 21 p.390]
<u>Purpose</u> – to increase intracranial venous drainage by affecting dural membranes that comprise the occipital, transverse and sagittal sinuses.[32 p.584]

B. <u>Compression of the fourth ventricle (CV4)</u>
<u>Purpose</u> – To improve motion of the C.R.I.[32 p.580] This is done by first resisting the flexion phase and encouraging the extension phase of the C.R.I. until a "still point" is reached, then allowing restoration of normal flexion and extension to occur.[28 p.169-70]

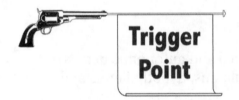

Trigger Point

The CV4 will improve motion of the C.R.I.

D. <u>V spread</u>
<u>Purpose</u> – To separate restricted or impacted sutures. The principle can be applied to any suture.[28 p.170]

E. <u>Lift technique</u>
<u>Purpose</u> – Frontal and parietal lifts are commonly used to aid in the balance of membranous tension.[28 p.170]

F. <u>Temporal Rocking</u>
<u>Purpose</u> – Treat dysfunction in which the temporal bone is held in external/internal rotation.[32 p.586]

VI. Indications for cranial treatment

Craniosacral treatment can be used for common strain patterns caused by any stresses that disturb the PRM. Craniosacral treatment can also be used in the following scenarios:[32 p.574]

1. Headaches
2. Whiplash
3. Vertigo and tinnitus
4. Otitis media with effusion and serous otitis media
5. TMJ dysfunction
6. Sinusitis

VII. Complications and contraindications to cranial treatment

A. Complications

Although uncommon, headaches, tinnitus, or dizziness has been reported following some treatments. SBS strain treatment may cause an alteration in heart rate, blood pressure, respiration, and gastrointestinal irritability.[32 p.575,1428 p.171]

B. Contraindications[32 p.574]

1. Absolute contraindications
   a. Acute intracranial bleed or increased intracranial pressure
   b. Skull fracture

2. Relative contraindications
   a. In patients with known seizure history or dystonia, great care must be used in order not exacerbate any neurological symptoms.
   b. Coagulopathies
   c. Space occupying lesions in the cranium

Chapter 9 Review Questions

1. A 20-year-old female presents with chronic headaches of 6 months' duration. Structural examination reveals a physiologic cranial strain pattern. The most likely diagnosis is

    A. inferior torsion
    B. left sidebending rotation
    C. right lateral strain
    D. SBS compression
    E. superior vertical strain

2. While palpating a patient's cranium with the vault hold you notice that the greater wing of the sphenoid feels more superior on the right than the left. You also notice that the occiput is rotated in the opposite direction. The most likely diagnosis is

    A. right torsion
    B. left torsion
    C. left lateral strain
    D. sidebending rotation left
    E. sidebending rotation right

3. A patient requests osteopathic manipulation for recurrent major depression that developed after a blunt injury to the front of the head. Structural examination reveals the CRI is virtually absent. The most likely diagnosis is

    A. lateral strain
    B. SBS compression
    C. sidebending and rotation strain
    D. torsion
    E. vertical strain

4. A 75-year-old female presents with chronic tinnitus. Which of the following strain patterns is most associated with this condition?

    A. ethmoid restriction interfering with CN IX
    B. sphenoid restriction interfering with CN VI
    C. sphenoid restriction interfering with CN X
    D. temporal restriction interfering with CN VII
    E. temporal restriction interfering with CN VIII

5. While palpating a patient's cranium using the vault hold you appreciate the extension phase of the primary respiratory mechanism. The motion of the paired structures will most likely undergo

    A. internal rotation
    B. extension
    C. symmetrical rotation
    D. flexion
    E. external rotation

6. While dissecting a cadaver you identify the superior and inferior attachments of the reciprocal tension membrane which consists of the

    A. base of the calvaria and the pelvis superiorly inferiorly
    B. base of the calvaria superiorly and thoracic inlet inferiorly
    C. inner surface of the calvaria, foramen magnum, C2, C3 , and S2
    D. thoracic inlet superiorly and the diaphragm inferiorly
    E. upper thoracic spine, ribs, and sternum superiorly, and the pelvis inferiorly

7. A 25-year-old female presents with chronic pelvic pain. Craniosacral examination reveals the sacral apex to be currently pushing into the palm of your hand. From this you can also state that the

    A. parietals are externally rotating
    B. occiput is moving into extension
    C. sacrum is moving into flexion around the middle transverse axis
    D. sphenoid is internally rotating
    E. temporals are moving into extension

8. A patient presents for osteopathic manipulation and a right sidebending rotation strain is diagnosed. Which of the following best describes this strain pattern?

    A. rotation about a vertical axis with both bones rotating the same direction
    B. rotation about an A-P axis with both bones rotating in the opposite direction
    C. sidebending about a vertical axis with both bones sidebending in the same direction
    D. sidebending about an A-P axis with both bones sidebending in the opposite direction
    E. sidebending about two vertical axes with both bones sidebending in the opposite direction

9. While assessing your patient's cranial rhythm using the vault hold, you note that the mechanism appears to easily allow your index fingers to move caudad while your little fingers move more cephalad. The most likely diagnosis is

    A. flexion dysfunction
    B. SBS compression
    C. midline torsion
    D. vertical strain superior
    E. lateral strain inferior

Questions 10-12 refer to the following:
   A young adult presents for a comprehensive sports physical before playing professionally. Vitals and physical examination are within normal limits. Structural examination with the vault hold reveals the midline bones to be in flexion.

10. This will cause the paired bones to undergo

   A. external rotation with a decrease in the anterio-posterior diameter of the cranium
   B. external rotation with an increase in the anterio-posterior diameter of the cranium
   C. internal rotation with a decrease in the anterio-posterior diameter of the cranium
   D. internal rotation with an increase in the anterio-posterior diameter of the cranium

11. Which of the following is most associated with this phase of craniosacral motion?

   A. deviation of the SBS caudad
   B. forehead becomes wide and sloping
   C. head lengthens in its anteroposterior diameter
   D. sacral base moves anterior and the apex moves posteriorly
   E. transverse diameter of the head narrows

12. The mastoid process of the temporal bones will most likely be

   A. anterior and medial
   B. anterior and lateral
   C. anterior and superior
   D. posterior and medial
   E. posterior and lateral

MATCHING
   For each numbered item (description) select one heading (cranial nerve) most closely associated with it. Each lettered heading may be selected once, more than once, or not at all.

   A. CN V1
   B. CN V2
   C. CN V3
   D. CN X
   E. CN XII

13. Exits the foramen rotundum.

   A. A
   B. B
   C. C
   D. D
   E. E

14. May be affected by somatic dysfunction of C2.

   A. A
   B. B
   C. C
   D. D
   E. E

15. Dysfunction may cause headache and an upset stomach.

   A. A
   B. B
   C. C
   D. D
   E. E

16. May become entrapped within the condylar part of the occiput.

   A. A
   B. B
   C. C
   D. D
   E. E

MATCHING
   For each numbered item (description) select one heading (manipulative technique) most closely associated with it. Each lettered heading may be selected once, more than once, or not at all.

   A. balanced membranous tension
   B. CV4 technique
   C. temporal rocking
   D. V spread
   E. venous sinus technique

17. Enhances intracranial drainage.

   A. A
   B. B
   C. C
   D. D
   E. E

18. Separates restricted or impacted sutures.

    A. A
    B. B
    C. C
    D. D
    E. E

19. A valuable technique to help TMJ dysfunction.

    A. A
    B. B
    C. C
    D. D
    E. E

20. Enhances the amplitude of the CRI.

    A. A
    B. B
    C. C
    D. D
    E. E

Explanations

1. Answer: **B**

    Physiologic strain patterns include right/left torsion (RT/LT) and sidebending rotation right/left (SBR_R/SBR_L) if their presence does not interfere with the flexion/extension motion of the primary respiratory mechanism. Flexion and extension are natural physiologic components of cranial movement and may also be considered a type of strain pattern if the mechanism does not move through flexion and extension equally.

2. Answer: **A**

    Torsions are named for the side of the high wing of the sphenoid and occurs around an AP axis of the skull.[1 p.737] In a torsion, the sphenoid of the anterior cranium rotates in one direction about this axis while the occiput and related structures of the posterior cranium rotate in the opposite direction. A twist or torsion at the SBS is produced.

3. Answer: **B**

    During SBS compression the basisphenoid and basiocciput are forced together which significantly limits motion of the sphenobasilar synchrondrosis (SBS) motion.[1 p.1108] The result is a decrease in the amplitude of the flexion and extension components of the CRI.

4. Answer: **E**

    The vestibulocochlear nerve (CN-VIII) has auditory and vestibular receptors in the petrous portion of the temporal bone. Dysfunction of the nerve may result in tinnitus, dizziness, or decreased auditory acuity. Treatment is aimed at releasing membranous strains of the cranial base, temporal bones, and upper cervical spine to re-establish synchronous motion.

5. Answer: **A**

    During extension the skull is long and narrow with temporals in relative internal rotation, frontals narrow with the brow appearing more vertical, orbits and face narrow, and maxillae narrow with a high arched vault.[1 p.739]

6. Answer: **C**

The reciprocal tension membrane includes the intracranial and spinal dural membrane including the falx cerebri, falx cerebelli, tentorium, and spinal dura. The calvaria is domelike superior portion of the cranium (skull cap), made up of the frontal, parietal, occipital and temporal bones. The dura firmly attaches to the inner surface throughout the cranium. The dura mater extends down the spinal canal with firm attachment around the foramen magnum and in the spinal canal of the sacrum at the level of S2. There are also two occasional attachments at C2 and C3 and the lower lumbar region.

7. Answer: **B**

This question has to do with the difference in motion of paired vs. midline bones. The sacral base (top part of sacrum) moves anteriorly and the apex moves posteriorly (into the palm of the examiner's hand) during the extension phase. This motion occurs around the respiratory axis – a transverse axis in the area of S2 posterior to the sacral canal (superior transverse axis). Cranial extension is also associated with narrowing of the cranium and extension of the midline bones (sphenoid, occiput, ethmoid, vomer), ascension of the top of the cranium, and internal rotation of all paired bones (i.e. temporals).

8. Answer: **E**

Sidebending/rotation at the SBS is a physiologic strain pattern that occurs around an AP axis and around two parallel vertical axes. The strain pattern is named for the side of the convexity (i.e. the direction the SBS deviated). The AP axis is the same as the axis around which torsions occur. The vertical axes are through the body of the sphenoid and another through the foramen magnum. However, unline a torsion, in this type of strain the sphenoid and occiput rotate in the same direction (see Fig. 9.6b). Sidebending occurs about two vertical axes (see Fig. 9.6a). Because the SBS is slightly convex upward, as the two bones sidebend away from each other causing the SBS to deviate to the right or left (around the two parallel vertical axes) both bones rotate inferiorly on the convex side (around the AP axis) and superiorly on the concave side.[1 p.737]

9. Answer: **D**

During the vault hold the index fingers are placed on the wings of the sphenoid (anterior to the transverse sphenoid axis) and the 5th digits are placed on the squamous portion of the occiput (posterior to the transverse occiput axis). The sphenoid and the occiput rotate in the same direction (either clockwise or counterclockwise) around their own transverse axes with vertical strains. This creates a superior or inferior strain at the SBS and disrupts normal flexion-extension movement, which is why this is not considered to be a physiologic strain pattern. It is named for the position of the sphenoid relative to the occiput: superior or inferior.

10. Answer: **A**

Palpation in the flexion portion of the biphasic cycle senses that the head widens slightly in its transverse diameter and shortens slightly in its anteroposterior (AP) diameter as the paired bones move toward external rotation. With extension of the midline bones, the head narrows and lengthens slightly, and all paired bones move toward internal rotation. During flexion, the sacrum moves posterosuperiorly at its base while the apex moves anteriorly toward the pubic bones.[1 p.735]

11. Answer: **B**

Questions like this bring out the nuances of cranial mechanics in a rule-out fashion. Midline bones move through flexion and paired bones move through external rotation thus causing the head to slightly widen and decrease in AP diameter. The forehead thus widens and slopes upward while the cheek bones widen. [1 p.739]

12. Answer: **B**

The mastoid processes are located on the inferior portion of the temporal bones. Paired bones externally rotate during flexion. During this movement the mastoid processes move laterally and anteriorly while the head slightly widens and decreases in AP diameter. See Figure 9.2 for a visual description.

13. Answer: **B**

The maxillary division of the trigeminal nerve (CN V2) courses through the inferior portion of the cavernous sinus, middle cranial fossa, foramen rotundum, pterygopalatine fossa, infratemporal fossa, and inferior orbital fissure.

14. Answer: **D**

There are well described vagal reflexes that tend to involve C2 due to extensive interconnections to cranial nerves and the C2 segment. The vagus nerve is responsible for referred pain and parasympathetic reflexes including posterior headaches referred from the throat, lung, heart, and bowel.[1 p.505, 20 p.58]

15. Answer: **D**

Dysfunction of the vagus nerve(CN X) may lead to referred pain and parasympathetic reflexes, headache, nausea, bradyarrhythmia, and cough.

16. Answer: **E**

The hypoglossal nerve (CN XII) is the motor nerve of the tongue. Entrapment nerve within the condylar part of the occiput caused by cranial dysfunction from birth trauma may result in difficulty suckling, dysphagia, and dysarthria.

17. Answer: **E**

The venous sinus technique increases intracranial venous drainage. Gentle hand contact on the external cranium influences the dura that comprises the venous sinuses. Release of the thoracic outlet should be performed prior to this technique. [32. p.584, 2 p.575]

18. Answer: **D**

V-spread is a technique using forces transmitted across the diameter of the skull to accomplish sutural gapping. This technique is performed by using a combination of disengagement and directing the tide.

19. Answer: **C**

The temporomandibular joint can be strained by a temporal bone held in external or internal rotation. This technique involves exerting pressure to find a point of ease between the bone's natural movement to release the restriction.

20. Answer: **B**

Compression of the fourth ventricle (CV4)enhances the amplitude of the CRI. It can beused to treat headaches, relieve sinus congestion, and reduce edema.[2 p.575]

Spinal Facilitation & Autonomic nervous system

10

I. Spinal Facilitation

<u>Definition</u> – the maintenance of a pool of neurons (e.g., premotor neurons, motoneurons of preganglionic sympathetic neurons in one or more segments of the spinal cord) in a state of partial or sub-threshold excitation. In this state, less afferent stimulation is required to trigger the discharge of impulses. Facilitation may be due to a sustained increase in afferent input, or changes within the affected neurons themselves, or their chemical environment. Once established, facilitation can be sustained by normal CNS activity.[1 p.1109]

A. <u>Neurophysiologic mechanism of facilitation</u>

If facilitation occurs at an individual spinal level it is termed segmental facilitation. In order to closely examine segmental facilitation we must first look at the spinal reflex. A spinal reflex is thought to have three simple parts:[34 p.65]

1. Afferent limb (sensory input)
2. Central limb (spinal pathway)
3. Efferent limb (motor pathway)

Unfortunately, this is an oversimplification. In actuality, sensory input originates from many places causing a variety of effects throughout the spinal cord. Within

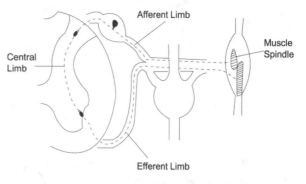

Fig. 10.1: *Simplification of a spinal reflex: Sensory input is transmitted by a afferent limb, processed by the central limb (interneurons) then a motor response is transmitted by the efferent limb.*

173

the spinal cord, ascending/descending, branching, and crossing interneurons process (and further complicate) the sensory information. Output at the spinal segment could be to lower motor neurons (dorsal/ventral rami) to muscle or to viscera via the autonomic nervous system. Thus, a spinal reflex is actually part of a vast ever-changing network of neurons that is finely tuned to regulate the activity of the body. [34 p.65]

B. How does a segment become (and stay) facilitated? (Figs 10.2 a,b)

A spinal cord segment can receive input from three areas:

1. Higher centers (brain)
2. Viscera via sympathetic or parasympathetic visceral afferents
3. Somatic afferents (muscle spindles, Golgi tendons, nociceptors, etc.)

Any abnormal and steady sensory stimulus from one of these three areas can cause the interneurons at a spinal cord level to become sensitive to the stimulus. These "sensitized" interneurons will have an increased or exaggerated output to the initiating site as well as other areas (neighboring muscles, or organs via autonomic efferents). Once the sensitized state is established, the segment is then considered to be facilitated. Any continuous sensitizing input or the presence of normal input through sensitized interneurons, will maintain the process and allow the abnormal situation to continue.

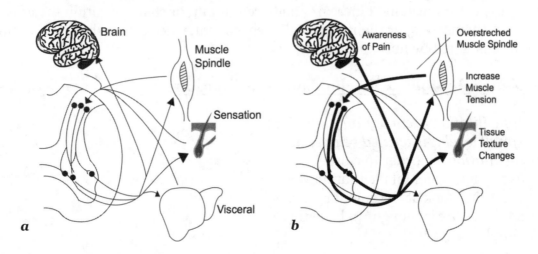

a   *b*

Fig. 10.2a: *Normal afferent and efferent circuit.*
Fig. 10.2b: *Facilitated segment: An abnormal sensory stimulus from an overstretched muscle spindle sensitizes two interneurons in the spinal cord. This will result in an increased or exaggerated output to the initiating site (resulting in increased muscle tension), as well as the brain (resulting in an awareness of pain), and local cutaneous tissue (resulting in tissue texture changes).*

C. **How does facilitation correlate with somatic dysfunction?**

Let us investigate what might occur when a patient strains his deltoid muscle.

1. Abnormal and continuous sensory input from the overstretched muscle spindle sensitizes the interneurons in the spinal cord at C5.
2. A reflex occurs so that muscle tension is produced at the deltoid muscle. This will result in a **restricted** range of motion of the deltoid and **tenderness** upon palpation.
3. Prolonged muscle tension causes continuation of the sensitizing input, and the maintenance of the facilitated segment.
4. Muscle tension at the initiation site (deltoid) causes nociceptor activation in the neighboring areas, and a release of bradykinins, serotonin, histamines, potassium, prostaglandins, substance P, and leukotrienes.[8 p.917] These substances will cause local vasodilatation and **tissue texture changes**.
5. The abnormal and continuous sensory input into C5 may also cause a paraspinal muscle spasm. The facilitated interneurons may cause an exaggerated motor output through the dorsal rami at C5 causing increased muscle tension in the deep paraspinal muscles. The resulting increase in muscle tension will cause C5 to rotate or sidebend so that **asymmetry** is present.
6. Therefore, a facilitated segment can lead to:

   1. **T**issue texture change.
   2. **A**symmetry.
   3. **R**estriction.
   4. **T**enderness.

   TART = the diagnostic criteria for somatic dysfunction.

D. **Reflexes**

1. Viscero-somatic reflex (Fig 10.3)

   According to the Glossary of Osteopathic Terminology, a viscero-somatic reflex occurs when localized visceral stimuli produce patterns of reflex response, in segmentally related somatic structures. For example, acute cholecystitis often refers pain to the mid-thoracic region at the tip of the right scapula.[1 p.1101]

2. Somato-visceral reflex

   Somatic stimuli may produce patterns of reflex response in segmentally related visceral structures. For example, a triggerpoint located in the right pectoralis major muscle, between the fifth and sixth ribs and just medial to the nipple line, has been known to cause supraventricular tachyarrhythmias.[1 p.1101]

Although viscero-somatic and somato-visceral reflexes are probably the most common, other reflexes are also possible. They include: somato-somatic, viscero-visceral, psycho-somatic, and psycho-visceral reflexes.

E. How does facilitation correlate with these reflexes?

Lets investigate how acute cholecystitis can cause referred pain to the mid-thoracic region at the tip of the right scapula, and somatic dysfunction of T5 - T9 (a common viscero-somatic reflex).

1. Continued gallbladder dysfunction, most often caused by gallstones, [22 p.926] will transmit an abnormal sensory input (from visceral receptors) into the spinal cord. This will result in segmental facilitation of T5 - T9.

2. Normal sensory input from general afferents (e.g., muscle spindle) at T5 - T9 will become amplified at the sensitized interneurons, resulting in an exaggerated motor response. This will cause an increase in tension in the paraspinal musculature of T5 - T9. Tenderness and pain can then be elicited at this region.

3. In addition, the increased muscle tension in the paraspinal muscles, will cause T5 - T9 to rotate and sidebend so that somatic dysfunction is present.

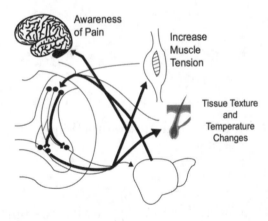

Fig. 10.3: *Viscero-somatic reflex: Continued visceral dysfunction will transmit abnormal sensory input into the spinal cord, resulting in facilitation of the interneurons. This will result in an exaggerated efferent response to somatic structures and the brain.*

NOTE: Another common viscero-somatic reflex is T1-T5 somatic dysfunction, and pain radiating into the jaw and left arm, associated with cardiac dysfunction.[1 p.121]

II. Autonomic innervation

Since visceral dysfunction transmits information to the spinal cord via autonomic afferents, it is essential for the osteopathic physician to understand the somatic areas likely to show effects of underlying visceral pathologic conditions through viscero-somatic reflexes. Table 10.1 demonstrates the effects of the autonomic nervous system on various organ systems. Fig 10.4 on the following page details the visceral innervation of the parasympathetic nervous system. Table 10.2 shows the visceral innervation of the sympathetic nervous system.

Table 10.1 [35] p.275, 36 p.250, 37 p.672, 29 pp. 38, 126, 127,188,

Structure	Parasympathetic Function	Sympathetic Function

Eye
    pupil
    lens
	Constricts (miosis)
	Contracts for near vision
		Dilates (mydriasis)
		Slight relaxation for far vision

Glands nasal, lacrimal, parotid, submandibular, gastric and pancreatic	Stimulates copious secretion	Vasoconstriction for slight secretion.
Sweat Glands	Sweating on palms of hands	Copious sweating (cholinergic)
Heart	Decreases contractility and conduction velocity	Increases contractility and conduction velocity

Lungs
    Bronchiolar smooth muscle
    Respiratory epithelium
	Contracts
	
	Decreases # of goblet cells to enhance thin secretions
		Relaxes
		
		Increases # of goblet cells to produce thick secretions

GI tract
    Smooth muscle
    lumen
    sphincters
    Secretion and Motility
	
	Contracts
	Relaxes
	Increases
		
		Relaxes
		Contracts
		Decreases

Systemic arterioles
    skin and visceral vessels
    skeletal muscle
	None
	None
		Contracts
		Relaxes

Genitourinary
    bladder wall (detrusor)
    bladder sphincter (trigone)
    penis
	Contracts
	Relaxes
	
	Erection
		Relaxes
		Contracts
		
		Ejaculation

Kidneys	Unknown	Vasoconstriction of afferent arterioloe => Decreased GFR => decreased urine volume
Ureters	Maintains normal peristalsis	Ureterospasm
Liver	Slight glycogen synthesis	Glycogenolysis (release of glucose into bloodstream)

Uterus
    body (fundus)
    cervix
	Relaxation
	Constricts
		Constricts
		Relaxes

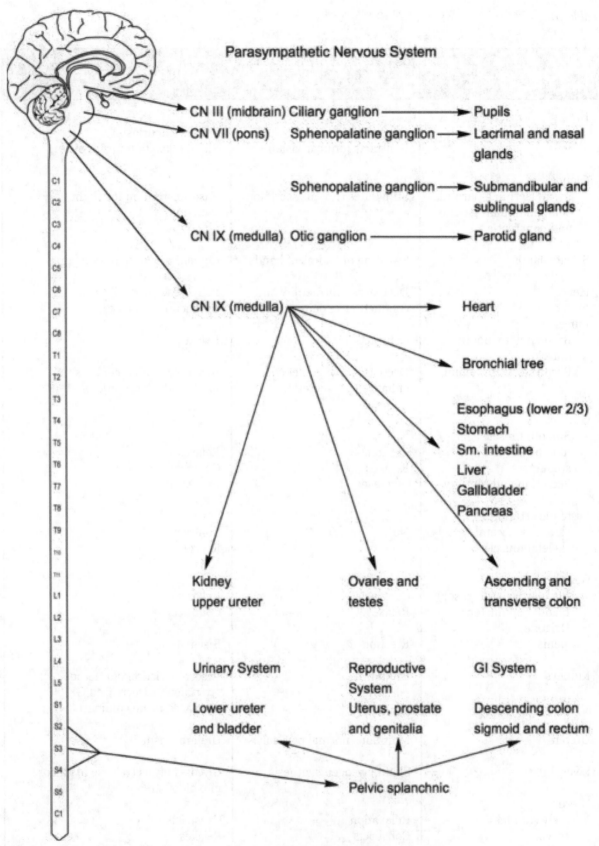

Figure 10.4: *Visceral innervation of the Parasympathetic Nervous System*

Sympathetic Nervous System

<u>NOTE:</u> Segmental sympathetic innervation varies from individual to individual and consequently will vary from author to author. There is no need to memorize the exact innervation for all the organs, but rather become familiar with the region of the spinal cord that innervates the viscera.

Table 10.2 [1 p.154, 32 p.485, 29 pp. 125, 192-3]

Visceral Organ	Spinal Cord Level	Corresponding Nerve and Ganglion
Head and neck	T1 - T4	
Heart	T1 - T5	
Respiratory System	T2 - T7	
Esophagus	T2 - T8	
Upper GI Tract	T5 - T9	
Stomach		Greater Splanchnic Nerve
Liver		Celiac Ganglion
Gallbladder		
Spleen		
Portions of the pancreas and duodenum		
Middle GI tract	T10 - T11	
Portions of the pancreas and duodenum		Lesser Splanchnic Nerve
Jejunum		Superior Mesenteric Ganglion
Ilium		
Ascending Colon & proximal 2/3 of transverse colon (a.k.a. right colon)		
Lower GI Tract	T12 - L2	
Distal 1/3 of transverse colon		Least Splanchnic Nerve
Descending colon & Sigmoid colon (a.k.a. left colon)		Inferior Mesenteric Ganglion
Rectum		
Appendix	T12	
Kidneys	T10 - T11	Superior Mesenteric Ganglion
Adrenal medulla	T10	
Upper Ureters	T10 - T11	Superior Mesenteric Ganglion
Lower Ureters	T12 - L1	Inferior Mesenteric Ganglion
Bladder	T11 - L2	
Gonads	T10 - T11	
Uterus and cervix	T10 - L2	
Erectile tissue of penis and clitoris	T11 - L2	
Prostate		
Extremities	T12 - L2	
Arms		
Legs	T2 - T7 [64 p.485]	
	T10 - L3 [64 p.485]	

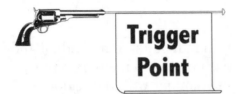

It is essential for anyone taking the COMLEX® boards to understand the segmental innervation to each visceral organ. Approximately 20% of the OMT boards questions will stem from Fig 10.4 and Table 10.2.

A. **Key points concerning autonomic innervations**

1. <u>Parasympathetic</u>

Most COMLEX®questions will test on which structures receive innervation from the vagus vs. the pelvic splanchnic.

<u>Here's an easy way to distinguish the difference:</u>
   - All viscera above the diaphragm = Vagus nerve
   - Below the diaphragm there are three main organ systems:

1) <u>GI system:</u>
   - Entire small intestine = vagus
   - Large intestine: There are four sections of the large intestine. Ascending, transverse, descending and recto-sigmoid. Divide the large intestine in half:
   Proximal half = Ascending and transverse = Vagus
   Distal half = Descending and recto-sigmoid = Pelvic splanchnic

2) <u>GU system</u>: There are three major structures. The kidneys, ureters and bladder (leave the urethra out of this it is not considered a major structure).
   Proximal half = Kidneys and upper ureter = Vagus
   Distal half = Lower ureter and bladder = Pelvic splanchnic

3) <u>Reproductive system</u>: The ovaries and testes descend from a higher region in the posterior abdominal wall, [5 p.145] therefore their innervations are from the vagus. All other reproductive structures are innervated by the pelvic splanchnic.

© Copyright 2018

2. <u>Sympathetic</u>
    a. <u>T1-T4</u> = Head and neck
    b. <u>T1-T5</u> = Heart
    c. <u>T2-T7</u> = Lungs
    d. <u>T5-L2</u> = Entire GI tract

An easy way to divide the GI tract
<u>Remember two landmarks</u>
1) **Ligament of Treitz** - divides the duodenum and jejunum
2) **Splenic flexure of the large intestine** - divides the transverse and descending colon

Anything before the ligament of Treitz = T5 - T9
Anything between these two landmarks is innervated by T10 - T11.
Anything after the Splenic flexure = T12 - L2
    e. <u>T2-T7</u> = Upper Extremities [32 p.485]
    f. <u>L3-L5</u> = **NOTHING!!**

III. Osteopathic manipulation directed at the autonomic nervous system

A. <u>Autonomic nervous system</u>

Irvin Korr, PhD (osteopathic researcher) established that there is hypersympathetic activity in disease processes. [7 p.73] Therefore, it is important to curb sympathetic activity (or enhance parasympathetic activity) when treating disease states.

B. <u>Sympathetic nervous system</u>

1. <u>Rib raising</u>
<u>Purpose #1:</u> *Normalize (decrease) sympathetic activity.*
    Since the thoracic sympathetic ganglia lie anterior to their corresponding rib, gentle anterior pressure on these ganglia will initially produce a short-lived increase in sympathetic activity, but this is followed by long lasting sympathetic inhibition.[7 p.57, 20 p.69]
<u>Examples:</u>
    1. Hypersympathetic activity to mucus membranes of the sinuses and the bronchial tree promotes the proliferation of goblet cells and produces thick, sticky, tenacious secretions. Rib raising to T2 - T7 will thin mucous secretions and thus enhance expectoration.[28.p.65]
    2. Rib raising and paraspinal inhibition reduced the incidence of an ileus in post-surgical patients from 7.6% to 0.3%. [7 p.76]

Purpose #2: *Improve lymphatic return*
Example:
    Since there is sympathetic innervation to the larger lymphatic vessels, rib raising will reduce vessel constriction and improve lymphatic return. In addition it will create pressure gradients directly affecting lymph return.[7 p.66, 32 p.148]

Purpose #3: Encourages maximum inhalation and provokes a more effective negative intrathoracic pressure. [29 p.195, 32 p.148]

Indications: [29 p.228, 20]
- Lower respiratory tract problems (pneumonia)
- Thoracic cage dysfunction/decreased rib excursion
- Lymphatic congestion
- Fever
- Paraspinal muscle spasm
- Congestive heart failure (CHF)
- Post-operative patient (improves rib excursion)

Contraindications: [29 p.228, 32 p.496]
- Spinal or rib fracture
- Recent spinal surgery
- Spinal cord injury
- Malignancy

2. Soft tissue paraspinal inhibition [29 p.198]
Purpose: *Normalize (decrease) sympathetic activity (ileus prevention)*
    The upper lumbar (L1 and L2) sympathetic ganglia is continuous with that of the thoracic paraspinal ganglia. However, due to the absence of ribs, direct paraspinal pressure on the erector spinae mass produces the same autonomic effects as rib raising. [7 p.57]

3. Celiac ganglion, superior mesenteric, inferior mesenteric releases
Purpose: *Normalize (decrease) sympathetic activity*
    Midline abdominal pressure over the celiac, superior mesenteric, and/or inferior mesenteric ganglia will reduce hypersympathetic activity. Pressure is applied until a fascial release is palpable. [7 p.76]

Indications: [29 p.227]
- GI dysfunction
- Pelvic dysfunction

Contraindications: [329p.227]
- Aortic aneurysm
- Open surgical wound

4. Treatment of Chapman's reflexes
   Purpose: Decrease sympathetic tone to associated visceral tissues
   Diagnose and treat Chapman's reflexes for visceral dysfunction.
   Chapman's points are treated using deep, firm, or gentale rotatory
   movement over the point itself.[1 p.857] Posterior Chapman's points feel
   rubbery, similar to a classic viscerosomatic reflex.

5. Treatment of cervical paraspinal sympathetic ganglia
   Treatment techniques adjacent to the superior (C1 - C3), middle (C6 -
   C7), and inferior (C7 - T1) ganglia may influence sympathetic tone to the
   head and neck structures. [7 p.58]

C. Parasympathetic nervous system

1. Cranial manipulation
   Purpose: Aids in dural strains and improves parasympathetic function in
   head structures innervated by CN III, VII, IX and X. [29 p.224]

2. Sphenopalatine ganglion technique
   Purpose: Enhancing parasympathetic activity will encourage thin watery
   secretions through short intermittently manual finger pressure intraorally
   to the sphenopalatine ganglion. [7 p.65]

   Indications: [29 p.231]
        - Thick nasal secretions

3. Decompression of the occipital condyles
   Purpose: Balance the reciprocal tension membrane (RTM) at the
   hypoglossal canal, permitting normal function of CN XII (Hypoglossal
   nerve). [32 p.578]

   Example: Condylar compression as a result of childbirth may cause
   suckling difficulties for the newborn and thus failure to thrive. [29 p.7] Treat
   this problem with condylar decompression.

4. Treatment through vagus nerve influence
   Purpose: Balance parasympathetic influence to the viscera. Manipulation
   of the OA, AA or C2 joints will influence parasympathetic tone via the
   vagus nerve. [1 p.506, 7 p.79, 29 p.224]

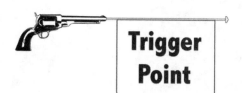

Trigger Point

Condylar compression may cause suckling difficulties for the newborn.

5. Treatment of sacral somatic dysfunctions
    Sacral rocking
        Purpose: [29 p.231, 32 p.497]
            1. Normalize hyperparasympathetic activity in the left colon, and pelvic structures.
            2 Improve SI joint mobility

        Indications: [32 p.497]
            - Dysmenorrhea
            - Pelvic congestion syndrome
            - Sacroiliac dysfunction

        Contraindications: [32 p.497]
            - Undiagnosed pelvic pain
            - Pelvic malignancy

Chapter 10 Review Questions

1. A male patient presents with indigestion and is found to have tissue texture changes along the posterior spinal column. It is determined that his symptoms resulted from somatic sensory stimulation with segmental spinal facilitation that is mediated through autonomic efferent nerves. This is a description of which of the following?

   A. central facilitation
   B. somatosomatic reflex
   C. somatovisceral reflex
   D. viscerosomatic reflex
   E. viscerovisceral reflex

2. A young female presents for osteopathic manipulation. During the structural exam a lesion at T3 is identified. Stimulation of the sympathetic chain ganglia at this region may contribute to

   A. bronchoconstriction
   B. detrusor contraction
   C. miosis
   D. lacrimation
   E. tachycardia

3. A 15-year-old male presents to your office with an acute asthmatic exacerbation. Structural examination will most likely reveal tissue texture changes at

   A. C2-C7
   B. T2-T6
   C. T5-T10
   D. T9-T11
   E. T12-L2

4. A teenage male presents to urgent care with an acute panic attack. The autonomic nervous system is most likely in sympathetic overdrive. This is associated with which of the following?

   A. glycogen synthesis
   B. increase in gastric motility
   C. increase in respiratory rate
   D. lacrimation
   E. miosis

5. A 42-year-old obese female presents with right upper quadrant pain that radiates to the tip of the right scapula. Examination reveals severe pain while the patient inhales with your fingers beneath the right subcostal margin. At which vertebral levels would you expect to find somatic changes?

    A. T1-T4
    B. T6-T9
    C. T9-T11
    D. T11-L2
    E. L1-L4

6. A viscerosomatic reflex resulting from a right colon cancer would be associated with somatic changes at which spinal segment?

    A. T5
    B. T8
    C. T11
    D. L2
    E. right tensor fasciae latae

7. A middle-aged male alcoholic presents with vague abdominal pain. Physical examination reveals scleral icterus, abdominal distension, and caput medusae. Sympathetic innervation to the pathologic organ passes through the

    A. celiac ganglia
    B. inferior mesenteric ganglia
    C. otic ganglia
    D. pelvic mesenteric ganglia
    E. superior mesenteric ganglia

8. A 75-year-old male presents to your office with urinary hesitancy and nocturia of 6 months' duration. Treatment to which of the following spinal segments will best alleviate his symptoms?

    A. T5
    B. T8
    C. T11
    D. L1
    E. S2

9. A 25-year-old female presents to your office with dysmenorrhea. Viscerosomatic reflex changes associated with uterine dysfunction may be at which spinal level?

    A. AA
    B. C7
    C. T12
    D. L4
    E. S1

10. A middle-aged male presents with epigastric discomfort and heartburn. Structural examination will most likely find tissue texture abnormalities at which of the following?

   A. a block mid-thoracic reaction which although bilateral tends to be right-sided
   B. C2, T3, and T5
   C. C2 with a block reaction fixed in extension from T5-T7
   D. C2 right, and T9 right
   E. right-sided thoracolumbar and sacrum

11. A teenage male presents with acute right-sided testicular pain. A Doppler ultrasound of the scrotum reveals testicular torsion. This is most associated with tissue texture changes at

   A. T7-T10
   B. T10-T11
   C. L2-L5
   D. L5-S1
   E. right iliac crest

Questions 12-14 refer to the following:
   A newborn receives a structural examination and a restriction of the occipitomastoid suture at the jugular foramen is identified.

12. This somatic dysfunction is most associated with

   A. constipation
   B. gastritis
   C. hemorrhoids
   D. stress incontinence
   E. tachycardia

13. Osteopathic manipulation is focused on stimulation of the vagus nerve. Treatment will most likely lead to:

   A. contraction of gastrointestinal sphincters
   B. decrease in gastric motility
   C. increase in contractility of the heart
   D. pupillary constriction
   E. urinary retention

14. Treatment is then focused on the occiput and atlas. This may affect which of the following visceral structures?

   A. adrenal gland
   B. bladder
   C. pancreas
   D. pituitary
   E. thyroid

Questions 15-16 refer to the following:
    A young female presents with periumbilical discomfort which later migrated to the right lower quadrant. She has an associated fever and is experiencing anorexia and nausea.

15. Which of the following spinal segments may alter the parasympathetic innervation to the diseased organ?

    A. AA
    B. C7
    C. T9-T12
    D. T12-L1
    E. S2-S4

16. An increase in the sympathetic tone to the abdominal cavity will result in an increase in

    A. gastric motility
    B. gastrointestinal absorption
    C. gluconeogenesis
    D. goblet cell secretions
    E. pancreas activity

Questions 17-18 refer to the following:
    A 45-year-old male presents for a follow-up blood pressure check. Past medical history is pertinent for paroxysmal hypertension secondary to an adrenal pheochromocytoma.

17. Structural examination will most likely reveal tissue texture changes at which spinal level?

    A. OA
    B. T8
    C. T10
    D. T12
    E. L2

18. Sympathetic stimulation of the involved segment may cause

    A. bradycardia
    B. ejaculation
    C. erection
    D. increased lymphatic drainage of the lower extremities
    E. pancreatic secretion

Explanations

1. Answer: **C**

   A somatovisceral reflex is when the soma (body) either activates or inhibits a visceral (organ) function through spinal facilitation. A common example would be vasoconstriction of local vasculature resulting from cold temperatures. The combination of these words (somato- and viscero-) can be changed to create various meanings based upon the relationship. The majority of osteopathic medicine, however, deals with viscerosomatic reflexes when considering diagnosis and treatment.

2. Answer: **E**

   The viscerosomatic reflex for the head and neck, heart, respiratory system, and esophagus correlates to T3. Stimulation of the sympathetic ganglia at this region may contribute to mydriasis (pupil dilation), vasoconstriction of glands, sweating, tachycardia, bronchodilation. Conversely, the distractors listed are related to stimulation of the parasympathetic nervous system.

3. Answer: **B**

   The viscerosomatic reflex for the respiratory system is T2-T7. Please refer to Table 10.2 for more information.

4. Answer: **C**

   The sympathetic system contributes to our fight or flight response and would be activated during a panic attack. Patients may experience tachypnea and tachycardia, pupil dilation (mydriasis), and bronchodilation. In order to have more energy, glycogenolysis is initiated rather than glycogen synthesis.

5. Answer: **B**

   This patient most likely has cholecystitis as evidenced by the positive murphy's sign in this obese forty-year-old female. The viscerosomatic reflex for the gallbladder, liver, stomach, duodenum, and portions of the pancreas is T5-T9. The corresponding nerve and ganglion is the greater splanchnic nerve and celiac ganglion.

6. Answer: **C**

The right side of the colon is the middle GI tract. The viscerosomatic reflex for this region is at T10-T11. The corresponding nerve and ganglion is the lesser splanchnic nerve and superior mesenteric ganglion.

7. Answer: **A**

This patient has either acute alcoholic hepatitis or decompensated alcoholic cirrhosis. The viscerosomatic reflex for the liver, gallbladder, stomach, duodenum, and portions of the pancreas is T5-T9. The corresponding nerve and ganglion is the greater splanchnic nerve and celiac ganglion.

8. Answer: **D**

This patient most likely has benign prostatic hyperplasia/hypertrophy causing lower urinary tract symptoms. The viscerosomatic reflex for the prostate is T12-L2.

9. Answer: **C**

The viscerosomatic reflex for the uterus and cervix is T10-L2. Please refer to Table 10.2 for more information. Parasympathetic influence is through S2-S4.

10. Answer: **B**

Gastritis or heartburn is associated with viscerosomatic reflexes at C2 left, T3 right, and T5 left. Dysfunction at C2 on the left is associated with vagal stimulation contributing to dysfunction of all viscera above the diaphragm. T3 on the right is associated with visceral dysfunction of the esophagus. Tissue texture changes at T5 on the left correlates to the stomach.[20 p.309]

11. Answer: **B**

The viscerosomatic reflex for the testes is T10-T11. Please refer to Table 10.2 for more information.

12. Answer: **B**

This question has the appearance of being difficult, however, if you have committed the viscerosomatic reflex table to memory you may have identified that this is a difference of parasympathetic reflexes from OA-C2 vs. S2-S4. Restriction at the occipitomastoid suture will contribute to somatic dysfunction at the OA which is known to have viscerosomatic reflexes for the following: heart, lung, upper and middle GI, liver, gallbladder, pancreas, and kidney. Therefore, the correct answer is either the only one related to parasympathetic overdrive of these body regions. For example, tachycardia is incorrect because parasympathetic viscerosomatic reflexes contribute to bradycardia for the heart. All of the other answer choices are associated with somatic dysfunction at S2-S4. On a related note, cranial nerves IX, X, and XI and the internal jugular vein pass through the jugular foramen.

13. Answer: **D**

Stimulation of the vagus nerve activates the parasympathetic nervous system. The vagus nerve innervates many organ systems above the diaphragm. Using this information we can rule out many of the answer choices. For example, parasympathetic stimulation of the gastrointestinal tract causes relaxation of sphincters and an increase in motility to promote digestion. Parasympathetic stimulation of the heart will slow down the heart rate and decrease contractility. The vagus nerve does not innervate the bladder or urethra, so we can rule out the urinary retention option.

14. Answer: **C**

The occiput, C1, and C2 are associated with parasympathetic viscerosomatic reflexes of several body regions including: heart, lungs, upper and middle GI system, pancreas, liver, gallbladder, kidney, and proximal ureter.

15. Answer: **A**

You should identify that this patient has acute appendicitis and then determine what parasympathetic viscerosomatic reflex is associated with this. The upper and middle GI system is mediated through the occiput, C1, and C2. The descending colon and rectum, however, is mediated through S2-S4. All of the other answer choices have to do with sympathetic viscerosomatic reflexes.

16. Answer: **C**

Sympathetic function of the gastrointestinal tract is associated with relaxation of the smooth muscle of the lumen, contraction of sphincters, and a decrease in secretions and motility. The sympathetic nervous system also stimulates gluconeogenesis of the liver and glycogenolysis to provide more available energy to cells and muscles.

17. Answer: **C**

The viscerosomatic reflex for the adrenal gland is T10. Please refer to Table 10.2 for more information.

18. Answer: **B**

The T10 spinal segment correlates to many body regions including the middle GI tract, kidneys, adrenal medulla, upper ureter, gonads, uterus, and lower extremities. Sympathetic stimulation of this segment may contribute to tachycardia due to activation of the adrenal gland, ejaculation due to activation of the gonads, decreased GI motility and secretions, and cessation of lymph flow to preserve energy.

Chapman's and Trigger Points

11

I. <u>Chapman's Points</u>

<u>Definition:</u>

    Starting in the early 1900's, Frank Chapman D.O. discovered that specific "gangliform contractions" were associated with visceral dysfunction. [38] These "gangliform contractions" were later called Chapman's reflex points or simply Chapman's points. These reflex points are *smooth, firm, discretely palpable nodules, approximately 2-3 mm in diameter, located within the deep fascia or on the periosteum of a bone.*[1 p. 855, 20 p.52] They often demonstrate sharp, pinpoint nonradiating tenderness. They are commonly located posteriorly in the tissues adjacent to the spine and anteriorly often in segmentally related tissues.[30 p.52] For a Chapman's reflex point to be positive, both the anterior and posterior points should be present. [1 p.855]

    Chapman's reflexes, in current clinical practice, are used more for diagnosis than for treatment. *They are thought to represent viscero-somatic reflexes.* **Therefore, a Chapman's point represents the somatic manifestation of a visceral dysfunction.** Palpating for a Chapman's reflex point can often provide the physician with clinical evidence of the presence or absence of visceral disease.

Table 11.1 [20] p. 58-63

Location	Anterior	Posterior
Upper respiratory tract	Near clavicle, rib 1 or 2	C1or C2
Lower respiratory tract		
Bronchi	Rib 2 and 3 at sternocostal junction	T2
Upper lung	Rib 3 and 4 at sternocostal junction	T3/4
Lower lung	Rib 4 and 5 at sternocostal junction	T4/5
Upper GI tract		
Esophagus	Rib 2 and 3 at sternocostal junction	T2
Stomach	Ribs 5-7 left	T5-7 (left)
Liver, gallbladder,	Ribs 5-7 right	T5-7 (right)
Pancreas	Ribs 7 and 8 at costocondral junction right	T7-8 (right)
Spleen	Ribs 7 and 8 at costocondral junction left	T7-8 (left)
Duodenum	Rib 8 and 9 near costocondral junction	T8,9
Jejeunum	Rib 9 and 10 near costocondral junction	T9, 10
Ilium	Rib 10 and 11 near costocondral junction	T10,11
Lower Gi tract		
Appendix	Tip of 12 right rib	TP's of T11/T12
Colon	See figure 11.1	L2-L4 to iliac crest
Heart	Between rib 2 and 3 at sternocostal junction	T2/3
Urinary system		
Kidney	1" above umbilicus either side of midline	T12, L1
Bladder	Periumbulcular and pubic symphysis	TP of L2
Urethra	Pubic symphysis	TP of L2
Reproductive system		
Ovaries/testes	Anterior pubic bone	T9-T11
Uterus	Medial border of obturator foramen	TP of L5
Prostate	Lateral femur (similar to colon)	TP of L5 to PSIS

In general anterior points are located at the sternocostal or costocondral junction unless otherwise specified in the table above, and posterior points are located between the spinous process and transverse process of the vertebrae. For example, if the table above states the posterior point is T2, that implies the Chapman's point is midway between the spinous process and transverse process of T2. Likewise T3/T4 implies between the transverse process of T3 and T4, midway between the transverse and spinous process.

To determine what portion of the colon corresponds to the Chapman's reflex, split the colon in the middle of the transverse colon and flip each side on to the corresponding iliotibial band.

The cecum point is located at the right proximal femur. The proximal transverse colon at the hepatic flexure is located at the right distal femur.

The sigmoid colon is located at the left proxima femur. The distal transverse colon at the splenic flexure is located at the left distal femur.

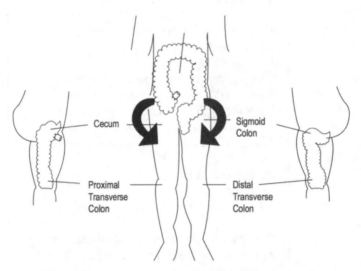

Fig 11.1: *Anterior Chapman's reflexes for the colon.*

MEMORY TOOL:

1) In general, an anterior Chapman point associated with a rib correspond to the same level as the thoracic vertebrae for the posterior Chapman point, except upper respiratory tract in which, rib 1 and 2 correspond to C1 and 2, respectively

2) Urinary system - anterior Chapman's points near umbilicus down to pubus and posterior T12-L2

3) Reproductive system - anterior on pubis and pelvis, posterior near L5 and iliac crest

II. Travell's Myofascial Trigger Points

A trigger point is a hypersensitive focus, usually within a taut band of skeletal muscle or in the muscle fascia. It is painful upon compression and can give rise to a characteristic referred pain, tenderness, and autonomic phenomena.[39 p.3]

A. Diagnostic characteristics

The patient may complain of tightness or soreness in a particular muscle that may or may not have followed an injury. On examination, the physician can palpate a taut band within the muscle. Upon compression of the band, the patient will experience pain at the site *and pain referring to an area of the body*. This referred pain is reproducible and specific for certain muscles. For example, trigger points located within the sternocleidomastoid will refer pain to occipital and temporal regions ipsilaterally. [39 p.7]

B. Pathophysiology

The spinal cord plays an important role in the establishment and maintenance of trigger points. Direct stimuli, such as a muscular strain, overwork fatigue, or postural imbalance, can initiate trigger points. This concept is very similar to facilitation. For example, if a person were to strain his deltoid, abnormal and continuous sensory input from the overstretched muscle spindle will sensitize the interneurons at C5. A reflex occurs so that muscle tension is produced within the deltoid at the initiating site, resulting in a taut band. If this taut band refers pain when compressed, then it is considered a trigger point.

Other stimuli, such as visceral dysfunction, may also facilitate the spinal cord (viscero-somatic reflex). For example, sixty-one percent of patients with cardiac disease were reported to have chest muscle trigger points.[39 p.586] Conversely, trigger points may facilitate the spinal cord and cause visceral dysfunction (somato-visceral reflex).[1 p.859] For example, a trigger point located in the right pectoralis muscle between the fifth and sixth ribs (intercostal space) near the sternum has been associated with supraventricular tachyarrhythmias.[40 p.577] **Therefore, a trigger point represents the somatic manifestation of a viscero-somatic, somato-visceral or somato-somatic reflex.**

C. Treatment

Myofascial trigger points can be treated in many ways. All techniques are directed toward eliminating the trigger point using a neurological or vascular method. The following procedures have been successful in eliminating trigger points: [40 p.9-10]

- Spray and stretch using vapocoolant spray
- Injection with local anesthetic or dry needling
- Muscle energy techniques
- Myofascial release
- Ultrasound, reciprocal inhibition, or ischemic compression

D. Trigger point vs. tenderpoint

Tenderpoints were first introduced by Lawerence Jones, DO Tenderpoints are small, hypersensitive points in the myofascial tissues of the body used as diagnostic criteria, and as a treatment monitor for counterstrain (Glossary of Osteopathic Terminology). Tenderpoints are similar to trigger points in that they are taut myofascial bands that are painful upon compression. *However, tenderpoints do not refer pain beyond the location compressed.* Some authors note a significant overlap in the location between trigger points and tenderpoints, [41] while some authors state that their distinction is somewhat arbitrary. [42]

Table 11.2[1 p.858]

	Chapman's points	Trigger Points	Tenderpoints
Location	Deep fascia/periosteum	Muscle	Tendon, muscle Ligament
Palpatory findings	Nodular, 2-3 mm to sizeof an almond	Taut Band	Discete, tense size of fingertip
Pain characteristics	Slightly painful to unbearable	Referred pain to predictible location	No referral of pain/ exquisitely tender
Association	Viscerosomatic reflex Rotary stimulation	Viscero-somatic, somato-visceral, somato-somatic	Somatic dysfunction
Treatment		See page 197	See Counterstrain

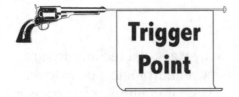

**Trigger points may refer pain when pressed.
Tenderpoints DO NOT refer pain when pressed.**

Chapter 11 Review Questions

1. A 42-year-old male presents to the emergency room with chest pain. He denies dyspnea, chest pressure of diaphoresis. Physical examination reveals his heart has a regular rate and rhythm with no murmers. Chest x-ray, EKG and cardiac enzymes are negative. Osteopathic structural examination reveals a group exhalation dysfunction of ribs 4-9 . A tenderpoint is located rib 4. Which of the following is most associated with the tenderpoint?

    A. acts a treatment monitor for counterstrain
    B. typically located in the deep fascia at the sternocondral junction
    C. pain is typically unbearable when compressed
    D. referred pain when compressed
    E. osteopathic treament consists of rotatory stimulation at the sight of the tenderpoint

2. A 10-year-old male presents with acute right lower quadrant pain. Physical examination is associated with acute abdominal signs. A ruptured appendix is suspected. Which one of the following Chapman's reflex points is associated with this condition?

    A. tip of the rib 11 on the right
    B. tip of the rib 12 on the right
    C. spinous process of L1
    D. spinous process of L2
    E. spinous process of T12

3. An elderly female presents for chronic constipation. Plain film radiography reveals distention of the ascending colon primarily. Structural examination will most likely reveal an anterior Chapman's reflex at which of the following?

    A. along the right iliotibial band
    B. at the left anterior superior iliac spine
    C. at the left pubic tubercle
    D. in the right lower quadrant of the abdomen
    E. two inches below the umbilicus

4. A 65-year-old has basilar pneumonia. The anterior Chapman point would be palpated

    A. in the intercostal space between the 2nd and 3rd ribs close to the sternum

    B. in the intercostal space between the 4th and 5th ribs close to the sternum
    C. in the intercostal space between the 6th and 7th ribs close to the sternum
    D. over the 2nd rib in the mid-clavicular line
    E. over the lateral mass of the atlas

5. Where should you palpate to find the anterior Chapman's tender point found in association with cardiac disease?

    A. in the 2nd intercostal space adjacent to the sternum
    B. in the center of the manibrium
    C. in the intercostal space between the 4th and 5th ribs at the sternocostal junction
    D. in the intercostal spaces between the 5th, 6th, and 7th ribs from the mid-mammillary line on the left to the sternum
    E. upon anterior aspect of the humerus at the level of the surgical neck

6. A 20-year-old female presents with nasal congestion, rhinorrhea, and maxillary sinus pressure ongoing for 2 weeks. The associated anterior Chapman's points for these regions are located in close proximity to the

    A. acromioclavicular joints
    B. clavicle near ribs 1 and 2
    C. middle third of each clavicle in the anterior cervical triangle (incorrect)n
    D. sternomanubrial joints
    E. xiphoid process

The following information pertains to questions 7-8:

An elderly male presents with shortness of breath and palpitations. An electrocardiogram is obtained and reveals a supraventricular tachyarrhythmia.

7. Structural examination will most likely reveal which of the following?

    A. crossover point at T6 left
    B. flattened thoracic kyphosis involving T5-T8
    C. Jones' anterior right rib 3 tenderpoint
    D. Travell's right pectoralis major myofascial trigger point
    E. lateral curve convex left

8. The tissue texture abnormality discovered is different from tenderpoints because this type

    A. is located in specific areas of the musculoskeletal system
    B. is located on the torso and never on the extremities
    C. is more tender when palpated
    D. results in pain perceived in a distant site called a reference zone
    E. usually lacks associated sympathetic dystonia

The following information pertains to questions 9-10

A teenager presents with chronic back pain. Structural examination reveals several Chapman's reflex points throughout the lumbar spine.

9. For a Chapman's reflex to be considered 'positive,' which of the following must be present?

    A. abdominal tenderness over the involved organ must be present
    B. both the anterior and posterior points must be present
    C. segmental somatic dysfunction must correlate dermatomally with the point
    D. the point must develop erythema when palpated
    E. the point must stay tender for more than 90 seconds after applying pressure

10. Which of the following best describes this type of somatic dysfunction?

    A. areas of cutaneous hyperemia that occur in response to visceral pathology
    B. areas of focally sympathetically-mediated sudomotor activity indicative of chronic visceral pathology
    C. distinct areas of tissue texture change specifically indicative of neoplasia
    D. palpable in soft tissue and demonstrate sharp, pinpoint, non-radiating tenderness
    E. segmentally specific myospastic contractions of paravertebral musculature

MATCHING

For each numbered item (patient presentation) select one heading (Chapman's reflex point) most closely associated with it. Each lettered heading may be selected once, more than once, or not at all.

    A. coracoid process
    B. midline of sternum
    C. proximal clavicle
    D. right 2nd intercostal space
    E. right 6th intercostal space

11. An obese 40-year-old female presents with right upper quadrant pain when she ingests fatty meals.

    A. A
    B. B
    C. C
    D. D
    E. E

12. A 14-year-old male reports ear pressure with associated dizziness.

    A. A
    B. B
    C. C
    D. D
    E. E

13. A 25-year-old smoker has frequent asthma attacks.

    A. A
    B. B
    C. C
    D. D
    E. E

Explanations

1. Answer: **A**

   Tenderpoints are small tense edematous areas of tenderness about the size of a fingertip.[1 p. 753] They are typically located near bony attachments of tendons, ligaments or in the belly of some muscles. Tenderpoints are monitored during counterstrain treatment. Trigger points are also a small, tense, hypersensitive areas of tenderness. However, trigger points will radiate pain to a specific area when compressed. Tenderpoints do not radiate pain to other locations of the body. Chapman's point are located in the deep fascia or periosteum and are associated with viscerosomatic dysfunction. Treatment of Chapman's points are

2. Answer: **B**

   The Chapman's reflex for appendicitis is the tip of rib 12 on the right anteriorly and the transverse processes of T11 and T12 posteriorly.

3. Answer: **A**

   The right or ascending colon corresponds to the right iliotibial band while the left or descending colon corresponds to the left iliotibial band. The cecum point is located at the right proximal femur, the proximal transverse colon at the right distal femur, the sigmoid colon at the left proximal femur, and distal transverse colon at the left distal femur.

4. Answer: **B**

   The anterior Chapman's reflex point for the lower lung is rib 4 and rib 5 at the sternocostal junction. The corresponding posterior points are at T4 and T5.

5. Answer: **A**

   The anterior Chapman's reflex point for the heart is located between rib 2 and rib 3 at the sternocostal junction. The corresponding posterior points are at T2 and T3.

6. Answer: **B**

   The anterior Chapman's reflex points for the upper respiratory tract are near the clavicle, rib 1, or rib 2. The corresponding posterior points are at C1 and C2.

7. Answer: **D**

A trigger point located in the right pectoralis muscle between the 5th and 6th ribs near the sternum has been associated with supraventricular tachyarrhythmias. There have been case reports of cessation of these rhythms with appropriate treatment of the associated trigger point.

8. Answer: **D**

The patient has a trigger point of the intercostal space between the fifth and sixth ribs causing SVT. Trigger points are the only type of tenderpoint which refer pain elsewhere in the body.

9. Answer: **B**

Technically both the corresponding anterior and posterior points should be present in order for to be considered a positive Chapman's reflex.

10. Answer: **D**

Chapman's reflex points are smooth, firm, discretely palpable nodules located within the deep fascia or on the periosteum of a bone. They are approximately 2-3 mm in diameter. They do not refer pain elsewhere in the body like Trigger points do.

11. Answer: **E**

This patient likely has biliary colic considering she meets the pathognomonic 'female, fat, forty, fertile' characteristic. The right sixth intercostal space is the Chapman's reflex point for the gallbladder and liver.

12. Answer: **C**

This patient probably has acute otitis media of the middle ear. The proximal clavicle is the Chapman's reflex point for the middle ear.

13. Answer: **D**

The right second intercostal space is the Chapman's reflex point for the bronchus as well as the esophagus, thyroid, and myocardium.

Myofascial Release

I. <u>Myofascial Release</u>

Myofascial release is a system of diagnosis and treatment first described by A.T. Still and his early students, which engages continual palpatory feedback to achieve release of myofascial tissues.[1 p. 1098, 32. 130]

This form of treatment combines several types of OMT in order to stretch and release muscle (myo) and fascia (fascial) restrictions. Counterstrain, facilitated positional release, unwinding, balanced ligamentous release, functional indirect release, direct fascial release, cranial osteopathy, and visceral manipulation are all forms of myofascial release.[21 p.380] Since counterstrain and facilitated positional release have unique features, they are discussed separately in Chapter 14.

Myofascial release treatment can be direct or indirect, active or passive (see Chapter 1, for a further explanation of these types of treatment). It also can be performed anywhere from head to toe, because fascia surrounds and compartmentalizes all structures throughout the body. For this reason, there are several different types of myofascial release techniques. It is not in the scope of this text to describe all of these treatments, but rather, a typical myofascial release procedure will be outlined.

A. <u>Typical myofascial release treatment</u> [32 p.132]

1. The physician palpates the patient with just enough pressure to engage the skin and subcutaneous fascial tissues. Then moves the tissues through x and y axes in order to determine the directionof restriction an direction of fascial ease (sometimes referred as a tight-loose or ease bind concept).[1 p. 707, 32 p.131] Occasionally the clinician may test the tissues in a clockwise/ counterclockwise relationship as well.

2. After determining the barriers, the physician must then decide the type of treatment (direct or indirect). This is often based on the clinical presentation and examination.[32 p.132]

    – *In a direct treatment, the physician will move myofascial tissues toward a restrictive barrier.*
    – *In an indirect treatment, the physician will move myofascial structures away from the restrictive barrier.*

    Occasionally, the physician can use a *combined technique*, where one hand approaches the tight barrier and the other the loose barrier. In addition, the physician may alternate between the tissues in a "neutral" point between the barriers (similar to functional technique). For more information of functional technique refer to Foundations of Osteopathic Medicine 3rd edition Chapter 52

3. Determine active or passive treatment. Once the myofascial tissues are engaged with respect to the desired barrier, the physican can then decide to use patient assistance (active treatment) or encourage patient to continue to relax (passive treatment). Some forms of active treatment ask the patient to perform isometric muscle contractions (clenching fists or jaw), tongue or ocular movements, or inhalation/exhalation. *These are generally referred to has "release enhancing maneuvers."* [32 p.131]

4. The physician then awaits a release. After approximately 20-30 seconds, a change in tissue compliance occurs. A release may come in many forms, a change in temperature, a tightness may "melt" or "give way." The release (aka fascial creep) may occur at different levels of the fascia or in several directions. The release phenomena is subtle and can only be appreciated by the skilled practitioner. Therefore, it may take several attempts before the osteopathic student can experience the release phenomenon.

5. The physician follows this change and continues to follow the fascial movement until no further evidence of creep occurs.

6. The physician reevaluates the tissues to determine if the fascial restriction has improved.

B. <u>Goal of myofascial release</u> [1 p.707]
In general myofascial release techniques help:

1. Restore motion in somatic dysfunction
2. Relieve edema
3. Relieve pain
4. Improve circulation and lymphy flow
5. Support visceral function

C. <u>Indications and contraindications</u>

<u>Indications</u>: Myofascial release techniques are typically gentle and can be performed on acutely ill hospitalized patients and elderly patients who cannot tolerate more aggressive therapy. Since these techniques can be done in multiple positions, they also can be done on those patients who cannot tolerate much movement.

<u>Contraindications</u>:[32 p. 132]

    <u>Relative</u>:
1. Acute sprain or strain
2. Fracture of dislocation
3. Neurologic or vascular compromise
4. Malignancy
5. Infection

    <u>Absolute</u>: none

Since myofascial release is a form of manual medicine that combines several types of OMT and has many applications, it is difficult to list specific indications and contraindications. It is important to remember that a goal of myofascial release is to improve lymphatic flow. Therefore, several of the indications and contraindications of lymphatic treatments can be applied to myofascial release techniques. For a list of indications and contraindications of specific myofascial release techniques, please see <u>Appendix A</u>.

II. <u>Fascial Patterns (Common Compensatory Patterns)</u>

Many authors have noted that the musculoskeletal system in most individuals is asymmetric J.Gordon Zink, DO was the first to provide documented material about these fascial preferences. Zink states that there are four compensatory curves throughout the spine: [1 p.796]

They are located at:

1. Occipitoatlantal junction
2. Cervicothoracic junction
3. Thoracolumbar junction
4. Lumbosacral junction

Rotatory testing of these segments reveal that in approximately 80% of **healthy individuals** the OA is rotated left, the cervicothoracic rotated right, the thoracolumbar rotated left and the lumbosacral rotated right. *Zink called this the Common Compensatory Pattern.* The remainder of **healthy individuals** (20%) had the opposite pattern. Zink called this the Uncommon Compensatory Pattern. He also noticed that unhealthy individuals, such as hospitalized patients, or those patients that recently experienced a traumatic event or stress, did not show this type of alternating pattern. In other words, their fascial preference did not alternate in direction from one reference area to the next. [7 p.46]

Table 12.1

Junction	Common Compensatory Pattern (80%) Rotation	Uncommon Compensatory Pattern (20%) Rotation
Occipitoatlantal	Left	Right
Cervicothoracic	Right	Left
Thoracolumbar	Left	Right
Lumbosacral	Right	Left

Chapter 12 Review Questions

1. A young male presents for a routine physical. Structural examination reveals he has the most common fascial pattern noted in the population. The most likely compensatory pattern is

    A. L / R / R / L
    B. L / L / R / R
    C. R / L / R / L
    D. L / R / L / R
    E. R / L / L / R

2. When performing indirect myofascial release, which barrier is engaged?

    A. anatomic
    B. elastic
    C. pathologic
    D. physiologic
    E. restrictive

3. Which of the following is an indication for treatment utilizing myofascial release?

    A. advanced stage cancer
    B. febrile bacterial infection
    C. osseous fracture
    D. peripheral edema
    E. traumatic disruption of internal organs

4. A young adult with chronic headaches undergoes osteopathic manipulative treatment. With the patient supine the physician holds cephalad traction to the suboccipital tissues until the regional musculature relaxes. This technique is a type of

    A. balanced ligamentous tension
    B. facilitated positional release
    C. Galbreath maneuver
    D. ligamentous articular strain
    E. myofascial release

5. A 38-year-old professional bowler presents with a chief complaint of intermittent numbness in the thumb and index finger. Physical examination reveals a positive Phalen test. Radiographs of the wrist are normal. The appropriate direct myofascial release treatment for this patient's includes

    A. stretching the flexor retinacululm
    B. increasing slack in the transverse carpal ligament
    C. circumduction of the wrist
    D. thumb adduction followed by gentle traction
    E. thumb flexion

6. You are consulted to see a severely debilitated 87-year-old male with complaints of mid thoracic pain. He was in the intensive care unit for 3 weeks and was transferred to a medical/surgical bed yesterday. He has a history of coronary artery disease, congestive heart failure and prostate cancer with vertebral metastasis. His back pain is localized to the mid thoracic region and seems to be musculoskeletal in nature. Which osteopathic manipulative techniques would be best suited to relieve this patient's symptoms?

    A. Muscle energy treatment with the spine extended
    B. Thoraco-abdominal diaphragm release
    C. High velocity low amplitude
    D. Pedal (Dalrymple) pump
    E. Direct myofascial release

7. A patient complains of neck pain that is worse at the end of the work day. Structural examination reveals somatic dysfunction in the upper cervical segments. The physician slowly turns the patient's neck in the direction of limited movement, loads the soft tissues with a gentle constant force, then waits a few seconds until the tissues release and more motion is possible. This technique is an example of

    A. articulatory technique
    B. counterstrain
    C. direct myofascial release
    D. facilitated positional release
    E. indirect myofascial release

Explanations

1. Answer: **D**

   This pattern is consistent with 80% of the general population. Zink noted that the natural homeostatic inclination was to develop an alternating pattern at the four transitional areas: OA rotating left, upper thoracic inlet rotating right, thoracolumbar junction to the left, and pelvis rotating to the right. The uncommon pattern has the opposite alternating fascial pattern.

2. Answer: **A**

   The anatomic barrier is the limit of passive (physician-mediated) motion. Movement to the point of the anatomic barrier is more comfortable and better tolerated away from the restrictive barrier. Indirect myofascial treatments move toward this direction. The physiologic barrier is the limit of active (patient-mediated) motion. The elastic barrier is a range between these two in which passive ligamentous stretching occurs before tissue disruption.

3. Answer: **D**

   Goals of myofascial release are to restore motion in somatic dysfunction, relieve edema and pain, improve circulation and lymph flow, and support visceral function. Osseous fracture, trauma malignancy and infections are relative contraindications

4. Answer: **E**

   Myofascial release engages continual palpatory feedback to achieve release of myofascial tissues. The tissues are loaded with a constant force until release occurs.

5. Answer: **A**

   The patient history and physical exam suggests carpal tunnel syndrome. The flexor retinaculum (tranverse carpal ligament) is a thickening of the deep fascia of the forearm and serves as the anterior wall of the carpal tunnel.[9 p.565] In a direct myofascial treatment the physician exerts tension on the carpal tunnel and stretches the flexor retinaculum.[32 p.143]

6. Answer: **E**

   Hospitalized patients typically respond better with indirect techniques or gentle direct techniques. Often these types of patients cannot withstand aggressive treatment. There are a variety of direct myofascial techniques that a physician can do that will not interfere with his fragile medical status. Muscle energy (regardless of the position of the spine) is contraindicated in patients with significant disabling medical conditions such as patients in the intensive care unit. Techniques geared toward improving lymphatic return are relatively contraindicated in patients with advanced stages of cancer. In addition, the thoracoabdominal diaphragm release and pedal pump are less likely to decrease this patient's mid-thoracic pain since it seems to be musculoskeletal in nature and not directly related to lymphatic congestion. High velocity low amplitude is contraindicated in patients with bone metastasis because this may cause a pathologic fracture to the spine.

7. Answer: **C**

Myofascial release engages continual palpatory feedback to achieve release of myofascial tissues. Direct treatments move into the restrictive barrier. The tissues are loaded with a constant force until release occurs.

Lymphatics 13

I. Overview:

The right upper extremity, the right hemicranium (including the head and face), and the heart and the lobes of the lung (except the left upper lobe) drain into the right (minor) lymphatic duct.[1] [p.791] Lymph from the remainder of the body empties into the left (major) duct. The thoracic duct traverses Sibson's fascia of the thoracic-inlet up to the level of C7 before turning around and emptying into the left (major) duct. The right (minor) duct only traverses the thoracic inlet once.[29 p.86, 210]

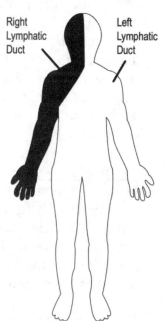

Fig 13.1: *The right upper extremity, the right hemicranium, and the heart and the lobes of the lung (except left upper lobe) drain into the right (minor) duct. Lymph from remainder of the body empties into the left (major) duct.*

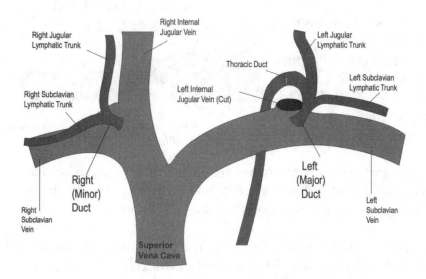

Fig 13.2: *The right (minor) duct drains into the right brachiocephalic vein. The left (major) duct drains the junction of the left internal jugular and subclavian veins.*

Since the thoracic duct transverses the superior thoracic inlet twice, the lymphatic system is particularly vunerable to fascial dysfunction at the thoracic inlet. Also, given the continguous nature of Sibson's fascia and the scalenes, scalene hypertonicity may impair lymphatic return.[1 p.792]

The lymphatic drainage of the right (minor) duct is variable; it usually drains into the right brachiocephalic vein or the junction of the right internal jugular and subclavian veins. The lymphatic drainage of the left (major) duct is more consistent; it drains into the junction of the left internal jugular and subclavian veins. Therefore, lymphatic drainage from an infection of the right first toe would drain into the left (major) lymphatic duct via the thoracic duct. A right maxillary sinus infection would drain into the right (minor) duct, as would extracellular fluid resulting from lymphedema of the right upper extremity.

II. <u>Anatomicophysiologic Relationships</u>

Lymphatic structures can be divided into lymphatic collecting systems and lymphoid tissue

<u>Lymphatic collecting symtems</u>
Lymphatics are tubes lined with endothelial cells, which drain the interstitium and viscera in general (Fig. 13.3). Lymphatic tubes drain into the initial collecting vessel, called a *lymphangion.*[1 p.193] Lymphagions contain one way valves that assist in moving lymph to larger pre-nodal vessels. Pre-nodal vessels lead to lymph nodes then onto larger post-nodal vessels.

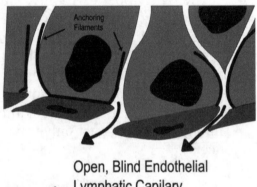

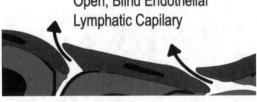

Fig 13.3: *Lymphatic fluid draining into a lymphatic capillary terminal.*

<u>Lymphoid tissue:</u>   (spleen, liver, thymus, tonsils, appendix, lymph nodes) are aggregates of lymphocytes and other immune cells.[43 p.1605] The spleen is the larges mass of lymphoid tissue in the body.[1p.790] One half to two-thirds of the lymphatic fluid is produced by the liver and intestines.[1 p.790, 37 p.180]

The thoracic duct extends approximately 18 inches from the cisterna chyli below the diaphragm (at the level of L2), through the aortic hiatus (at the level of T12) into the neck for about 3 centimeters before draining into the left (major) duct.[35 p.86]

Embryologically, the lymphatic system is developed by the third month in utero and the lymph vessels are closely related to the development of the venous system. Lymphoid tissue increases until 6-9 years of age. At puberty, the immune system matures and lymphoid tissue regresses until 15-16 years of age. Lymph tissue and function remain stable throughout most of adulthood. In ther geriatric patient, the system may decline to the point where the patient cannot amount a response (fever).

III. Function of Lymph

1) Purification/cleaning of tissues
   The lymphatics cleanse the body of immune complexes, bacteria, viruses, salts and 50% of the plasma proteins. Substances found in the lymph include amino acids, glycerol and glucose [21 p.256]
2) Maintaining fluid balance
   Approximately 10-20% of extracellular tissue fluid is carried from the interstitium to the blood circulation. This translates into at least 3 liters of fluid per day. [1 p.789, 43 p.1605]
3) Defense/immunology
   The lymphatics carry partulate waste, exudates and bacteria for the body's removal. They also are responsible for carrying antigens to the lymph nodes where the immune response is initated
4) Nutrition
   Vital to one's nutritional state, the intestinal lymphatics absorb long chain fats, chylomicrons, and cholesterol. [1 p.789]

IV. Innervation of Lymphatic System

It is important to realize that the lymphatic capillary is under the same sympathetic influences as are other vasculature. The sympathetics constrict the lymphatic capillaries. Initially, this will lead to an increase in peristalsis of the lymph vessel. However, sustained inappropriate hypersympathetic tone may decrease the overall movement of lymphatic fluids. Although there are cholinergic fibers in the lymphatics, little is known of the parasympathetic influence upon the lymph movement.

V. Factors Influencing Lymphatic Fluid Movement:

The lymphatics relieve the body's excess fluids and wastes by both intrinsic and extrinsic forces.

Extrinsic forces include:
   -Osteopathic manipulative treatment
   -Exercise
   -Contraction of muscles [43 p.1606]
   -Pulsation of adjacent arteries [43 p.1606]
   -Respiratory movement to increase negative intrathoracic pressure [43 p.1606]

Intrinsic forces include:
    -Smooth muscle contraction (controled by sympathetics) [43 p.1606]
    -Interstitial fluid pressure

Interstitial fluid pressure is normally -6.3mmHg and flows at a rate of 120cc/hr. Any increase of interstitial fluid pressure will increase the absorption of lymph into lymph capillaries. An increase to 0mmHg will increase lymph flow twenty-fold.[8 p.945] However at levels above 0mmHg interstitial fluid pressure becomes so great that it causes the lymphatic capillaries to collapse. As a result, there is a decrease in lymphatic drainage.

Factors allowing extracellular fluid to enter the lymphatic capillary:[37 p.182]
    1. Increased arterial capillary pressure.
    2. Decreased plasma colloidal osmotic pressure.
    3. Increased protein in the interstitium.
    4. Increased capillary permeability.

Factors increasing interstitial pressure above 0mmHg that correlate to numbers 1-4 above: [8 p.945]
    1. Systemic hypertension.
    2. Cirrhosis (decreased plasma protein synthesis).
    3. Hypoalbuminemia associated with starvation.
    4. Toxins such as rattlesnake poisoning.

VI. Osteopathic Diagnosis for Lymphatic Dysfunction:[29p.206]

1. Supraclavicular fullness and bogginess resulting from lymphatic congestion of the head and neck, e.g., sinusitis.
2. Posterior axillary fold fullness and bogginess resulting from lymphatic congestion of the arm, e.g., post-mastectomy lymphedema.
3. Epigastric area fullness and bogginess resulting from organ congestion of the chest or abdomen, e.g., cirrhosis.
4. Inguinal area fullness and bogginess resulting from lymphatic congestion of the lower extremity, e.g., infection.
5. Popliteal area fullness and bogginess resulting from lymphatic congestion of the leg, e.g., thrombophlebitis.
6. Achilles tendon fullness and bogginess resulting from lymphatic congestion of the ankle or foot, e.g., sprained anterior talofibular ligament.

Additionally, many other areas of dysfunction may lead to lymphatic congestion.
Some of these include:

7. Tense pelvic diaphragm (levator ani and coccygeus muscles).
8. Restricted thoracic cage motion [21 p.258]
9. Viscerosomatic tissue texture changes (Chapman's reflexes) from lymphatic congestion of any organ.
10. Paravertebral muscle spasm causing an increased lumbar lordosis with resultant flattened diaphragm.
11. Torsioned thoracic-inlet.
12. Cranial base strain, particularly along the attachments of the tentorium cerebelli (occiput, parietals, temporals, sphenoid or ethmoid).

VII. <u>Osteopathic Treatment for Lymphatic Dysfunction</u>

1. <u>Chapman's reflexes</u>
    Lymphatic congestion of the lower respiratory tract may produce a Chapman's point at ribs 2-5 nears the sternocostal junction or posteriorly between the spinous and transverse processes of T2, T3, T4 or T5. There are about 100 recorded Chapman's reflexes in the body.

2. <u>Thoracic pump (of Miller)</u>
    This facilitates increased rib cage motion in addition to mobilizing total lymphatic fluid movement.

3. <u>Pedal pump (of Dalrymple)</u>
    Again, this encourages total body lymphatic movement and is particularly useful for the pediatric patient.

4. <u>Osteopathy in the cranial field</u>
    This will decrease dural strains of what is considered the uppermost diaphragm of the body, the tentorium cerebelli and the reciprocal tension membrane in general. This will also increase venous return from the head by undoing strains at the occipital and temporal regions, which make up the jugular foramen (occipitomastoid suture). In addition, the CSF not only is considered the lymphatic fluid of the brain but also drains directly into the facial and spinal lymphatics.

5. <u>Muscle energy or any treatment to the thoracic-inlet</u>
    Remember Sibson's fascia is made up of the connective tissues of the scalenes and longus colli muscle and is traversed by both right and left lymphatic ducts.

6. Rib raising
   This will increase thoracic motion by lessened somatic dysfunction of the spine, ribs and sternomanubrial-clavicular complex. Also, normalization of the parathoracic sympathetic ganglia are achieved by rib raising.

7. Splenic/Liver pump
   This facilitates bringing toxins and other antigens into close contact with the macrophages of the liver (Kupffer cells) and allows the spleen to screen and remove damaged cells form the circulation [21 p.258]

8. Facial sinus pressure/Galbreath technique
   This includes direct "stroking" of the frontal, nasal, maxillary and zygomatic bones and/or the tempomandibular joint (TMJ) in order to facilitate lymph movement toward the jugulodigastric node (just anterior to the TMJ) and eventually distally to the right and left lymphatic ducts. This is useful in sinus congestion or otitis media.

9. Anterior cervical mobilization
   Basically, gentle translatory (right to left, vice versa) motion of the hyoid, thyroid, cricoid and trachea will also encourage lymphatic drainage of the head, neck and throat.

10. Extremity pump (of Wales)
    Involves effleurage wave-like motions of the arms and legs in order to move lymph proximally to the axillae and groin respectively before terminating into the right and left lymphatic ducts.

VIII. <u>Sequencing of Lymphatic Treatments</u>

Lymphatic treatments can be divided into two catagories. Those that improve restrictions and those that augment lymphatic flow. Treatment protocols should include techniques from both catagories. First start with techniques that remove restriction, then apply techniques that augment flow. [1] p.799 A basic sequence for lymphatic treatment program should include:

1. Open myofascial pathways at these transition areas of the body first:
   Four key transition sites (as popularized by Zink - see Chapter 12) are:

       Craniocervical junction
       Cervicothoracic junction
       Thoracolumbar junction
       Lumbopelvic junction

2. Maximize normal diaphram movement
"Redome" thoracoabdominal diaphragm and/or ischiorectal fossa release for pelvic diaphragm. This will optimize pressure gradients to maximize lymph return.

3. Apply lymphatic pump techniques
Once the diaphragms are free of restriction and sympathetic tone is normalized. Lymphatic pumps will help return lymph through open channels. Most pumps are performed at a rate of 120 beats/min for 2 min. [1 p.804]

4. Mobilize targeted tissue fluids into lymphaticovenous system
After the pathways are open, the practitioner may select to use techniques that decongest specifically targeted tissues, such as the posterior axillary fold technique for drainage of the upper extremity or the Galbreath technique for drainage of the head ande neck. [1 p.802]

IX. Indications for Lymphatic Treatment [1 p.793]

1. Acute somatic dysfunction
2. Sprain/strains
3. Edema, tissue congestion, or lymphatic/venous statsis
4. Pregnanacy
5. Infection
6. Inflammation
7. Pathologies with signifucant venous and/or lymphatic congestion

X. Contraindications to Lymphatic Treatment

The distinction between relative and absolute contraindications to lymphatic technique are unfortunately not well delineated. In fact, the Foundations of Osteopathic Medicine, 3rd Ed. only lists anuria or in an area of necrotizing fascitis as absolute contraindications. [1.p 793] To shed some clarity on the situation, the following lists are mostly extrapolated from the Foundations of Osteopathic Medicine 3rd Ed. [1 p.796] and An Ostopathic Approach to Diagnosis and Treatment. [2 p.591]

Relative contraindications to lymphatic treatment: [1 p.796, 2 p591]
1. Osseous fractures.
2. Certain circulatory disorders (venous obstructions, embolism, hemmorage)
3. Bacterial infections with a temperature greater than 102°F.
4. Certain stages of carcinoma.
   NOTE: This fact has not been demonstrated. Dowling argues that a case can be made for the delivery of cancerous cells to the body's immune system for clearance and destruction. [2 p.591]

Absolute Contraindication for lymphatic treatment: [1 p.793]
1. anuria
2. necrotizing fasictis

For contraindications to specific lymphatic treatments see <u>Appendix A</u>.

Chapter 13 Review Questions

1. A post-doctoral researcher is studying the drainage of lymphatic fluid with radionucleotide imaging in attempts to identify the structures which drain into the left (major) duct. Results of the study will most likely reveal fluid coming from the

    A. myocardium
    B. right eye
    C. right hemicranium
    D. right leg
    E. right upper lobe of the lung

2. Restrictions within Sibson's fascia could produce edema in

    A. both lower extremities
    B. head and neck structures
    C. the entire body
    D. the left upper and both lower extremities
    E. the right upper extremity

3. A patient presents with generalized edema and requests osteopathic therapy. With the hands around the thoracic cage and underneath the costal margin, the physician holds the facial tissues during patient inhalation and exhalation. This technique is called the

    A. facilitated positional release
    B. rib raising
    C. thoraco-abdominal diaphragm release
    D. thoracic inlet release
    E. thoracic outlet release

4. A patient presents with a mild viral syndrome. Home symptomatic care is recommended in conjunction with osteopathic manipulative treatment. Which of the following correctly outlines the correct typical sequence for lymphatic treatment?

    A. thoraco-abdominal diaphragm release, thoracic inlet release, lymphatic pump
    B. lymphatic pump, thoraco-abdominal diaphragm release, thoracic inlet release
    C. thoraco-abdominal diaphragm release, lymphatic pump, thoracic inlet release
    D. thoracic inlet release, thoraco-abdominal diaphragm release, lymphatic pump
    E. thoracic inlet release, lymphatic pump, thoraco-abdominal diaphragm release

5. In an attempt to facilitate lymphatic return to the thorax, prior to attempting lymphatic pump techniques, the physician should

    A. articulate the sternal angle
    B. articulate the sternocostal joints
    C. measure diaphragmatic excursion
    D. treat peripheral restrictions
    E. treat thoracic inlet restrictions

6. Respiration causes lymphatic movement centrally by the creation of

    A. negative intrathoracic pressure during exhalation
    B. negative intrathoracic pressure during inhalation
    C. positive intrathoracic pressure during exhalation
    D. positive intrathoracic pressure during inhalation
    E. thoracic duct smooth muscle spasms

7. A 65-year-old diabetic presents with cellulitis of the lower extremity. Lymphatic treatment using the popliteal spread technique is applied. The primary objective of this treatment is to

    A. Release restrictions in the popliteal fossa
    B. Decrease restrictions in the joint capsule of the knee
    C. Loosen medial and lateral collateral ligaments
    D. Release the gastrocnemius through effluage
    E. Normalize the sympathetic tone of the popliteal artery

8. A middle aged female presents with body aches, fever, and head congestion. She is assessed as having influenza and osteopathic manipulative treatment is provided. During treatment the physician utilizes the elastic recoil of the thoracic cage to create an abrupt change in intra-thoracic pressure. What is the most appropriate name of this technique?

    A. redoming the diaphragm
    B. indirect rib release
    C. pectoral traction
    D. thoracic lymphatic pump of Miller
    E. pedal fascial lymphatic pump

9. Pectoral traction affects lymphatic flow because the

    A. anterior axillary fold is directly released
    B. cisterna chyli is massaged
    C. clavicles are articulated
    D. posterior axillary fold is directly released
    E. sternum is released using the hypothenar eminence

10. The Galbreath technique is useful for treating those with

    A. bacterial conjunctivitis
    B. exudative tonsillitis
    C. nasal polyposis
    D. recurrent otitis media
    E. trigeminal neuralgia

11. A manipulative treatment that involves physician contact at the patient's supraorbital, mental, and infraorbital foramina is

    A. anterior cervical counterstrain
    B. frontal lift
    C. pterygoid fossa decongestion
    D. sinus inhibitory pressure
    E. vomer pump technique

12. A 40-year-old female presents with chronic chest discomfort. Structural examination reveals a severe restriction to the right thoracic inlet. Which of the following is most likely to have inadequate lymphatic homeostasis in this patient?

    A. cisterna chyli
    B. right lower extremity
    C. right lumbar lymphatic trunk
    D. right upper extremity
    E. small intestine and ascending colon

13. Which of the following structures is considered to be a physiologic diaphragm?

    A. broad ligament of the uterus
    B. greater omentum
    C. hard and soft palate
    D. mediastinum
    E. tentorium cerebelli

14. Thoracic inlet myofascial release would be useful for a patient who has

    A. functional scoliotic curve
    B. inhalation dysfunction of rib 6
    C. sacroiliac restriction with a tight piriformis muscle
    D. thoracolumbar extended dysfunction
    E. upper respiratory infection, tight scalenes, and rib 1 dysfunction

Explanations

1. Answer: **D**

   The right upper extremity, right hemicranium, heart, and most lobes of the lungs (except the left upper lobe) drain into the right (minor) duct. The remainder of the body drains into the left (major) duct.

2. Answer: **C**

   Sibson's fascia is comprised of connective tissues of the scalenes and longus colli muscle. It is also traversed by both the right and left lymphatic ducts. Therefore, restriction of Sibson's fascia can cause lymphedema of the entire body since both the right and left ducts are involved.

3. Answer: **C**

   The provider is grasping the patient around the thoraco-abdominal diaphragm. This procedure is used to relax the diaphragm and increase respiratory excursion thus maximizing lymphatic return.

4. Answer: **D**

   The recommended sequence of lymphatic treatment is primarily based upon protocols of various randomized control trials which were designed with the theory that we should first remove fascial restrictions and then apply techniques that augment lymphatic flow. The typical protocol includes opening myofascial pathways at transition areas (thoracic inlet release), maximizing normal diaphragm movement (thoraco-abdominal diaphragm release), applying lymphatic pumps then mobilize targeted tissue fluids into the lymphaticovenous system.

5. Answer: **E**

   The recommended sequence of lymphatic treatment is primarily based upon protocols of various randomized control trials which were designed with the theory that we should first remove fascial restrictions and then apply techniques that augment lymphatic flow.

6.   Answer: **B**

Inhalation causes negative intrathoracic pressure. Due to physics air tends to move into regions of lower pressure. The same physics apply to the fluids of our body.

7.   Answer: **A**

This is a form of direct myofascial release of the lower extremity. It is indicated to improve lymphatic and venous drainage from the lower extremities (knee, ankle, foot). [32 p.540] This technique does so by releasing fascial restrictions of the popliteal fossa.

8.   Answer: **D**

The thoracic pump of Miller facilitates an abrupt increase in rib cage motion to mobilize lymphatic fluid. In the supine position, the patient is instructed to exhale repeatedly while the provider increases resistance on the anterior superior chest. During a final inhalation the resistance is removed, forcibly causing an abrupt negative in intra-thoracic pressure. [32 p.520]

9.   Answer: **A**

Pectoral traction is intended to enhance motion of the diaphragm. With the patient in the supine position the physician applies cephalad traction beneath the anterior axillary folds. The patient is then instructed to breath deeply several times. The traction tends to pull the anterior thoracic cage into position of inhalation; in order to breath deeply the patient must better employ the motion of the thoracoabdominal diaphragm, thereby reducing restrictions and enhancing lymphatic flow.

10. Answer: **D**

The Galbreath technique involves direct slow rhythmic force of the mandible in a downward and transverse direction with the intent of repeatedly opening the Eustachian tube to allow the middle ear to drain accumulated fluid more effectively. Although it is indicated for any dysfunction of lymph in the ENT or submandibular region, it is especially useful in the dysfunction of the eustachian tubes. [32 p.511]

11. Answer: **D**

Sinus inhibitory pressure involves direct stroking of the frontal, nasal, maxillary, and zygomatic bones in order to facilitate lymph movement toward the jugulodigastric node and distally to the right and left lymphatic ducts. It is very useful for sinus congestion and otitis media.

12. Answer: **D**

The right upper extremity, right hemicranium, heart, and most lobes of the lungs (except the left upper lobe) drain into the right thoracic duct. The remainder of the body drains into the left (major) thoracic duct.

13. Answer: **E**

The four diaphragms of the body include the tentorium cerebelli, thoracic inlet, abdominal diaphragm, and pelvic diaphragm.

14. Answer: **E**

The thoracic inlet is in the upper chest and neck. If this is constricted it can prohibit lymphatic flow from the head and neck. Alleviating this constriction is often one of the first osteopathic manipulative treatments provided to those with upper respiratory infections in order to then mobilize lymphatic by other means.

Counterstrain and Facilitated Positional Release (FPR)

Counterstrain

I. Definition

*Counterstrain is a **passive indirect technique** in which the tissue being treated is positioned , away from the restrictive barrier.*[1 p. 749] Counterstrain was pioneered by Lawerence H. Jones in 1955. Jones discovered that by placing a patient in a position of ease for 90 seconds he could eliminate "tenderpoints." This treatment is now called counterstrain.[1 p.749]

A. What is a tenderpoint?
Tenderpoints are small tense edematous areas of tenderness about the size of a fingertip.[1 p. 753] They are typically located near bony attachments of tendons, ligaments or in the belly of some muscles. Trigger points are also a small, tense, hypersensitive areas of tenderness. *However, trigger points will radiate pain to a specific area when compressed. Tenderpoints do not radiate pain to other locations of the body.*

B. Basic counterstrain treatment steps

1. Locate a significant tenderpoint.
   – Tenderpoints are typically located in tendinous attachments or in the belly of the muscle. A significant tenderpoint is about four times more tender than the adjacent tissues. The pressure to elicit a tenderpoint is typically a few ounces (about the amount needed to blanch a fingernail of the palpating finger).[1 p.753] It is important to find the most significant tenderpoint associated with that somatic dysfunction rather than finding a point that is tender.[1 p.753]

    – Tenderpoints can usually be found at the region of the patient's chief complaint. In addition, tenderpoints may also be located in a corresponding anterior location.

    – Also keep in mind that pain at one location may be induced from a primary strain elsewhere. A common example of this is a patient with a psoas spasm complaining of low back pain. Although tenderness can be elicited at the lumbar spine and sacroiliac regions, a psoas tenderpoint located medial to the ASIS or periumbilical region will be present, and may be the cause of the lumbosacral pain.

2. <u>Establish a tenderness scale</u>
    – The most common method to establish a tenderness scale is 1-10. This provides the physician feedback for monitoring the efficacy of treatment.
    – The same amount of pressue should be used each time the physician assess for tenderness although different amounts of pressure is needed for different tenderpoints.

3. <u>Place the patient in the position of optimal comfort.</u>
    – Maintaining light contact with the tenderpoint, the physician makes a gross adjustment, **shortening the muscle** being treated.
    – Reapply firm pressure to check for reduction of tenderness.
    – Fine tune the treatment with small areas of motion until at least 70% (preferably 100%) of the tenderness has been reduced.[1 p.754]

4. <u>With the patient completely relaxed, maintain the position of comfort for 90 seconds.</u>
    – Ninety seconds is the time required for the proprioceptive firing to decrease in frequency and amplitude.[21 p.88-9]

5. <u>Slow return to neutral.</u>
    – The first few degrees are the most important.[1 p. 756]
    – Make sure the patient is completely relaxed and does not try to help by actively moving.

6. <u>Recheck the tenderpoint.</u>
    – No more than 30% of the tenderness should remain.
    – Tenderness from a viscerosomatic reflex will return within a few hours. [1 p.753]

II. Counterstrain Techniques

A. Cervical Spine

Anterior Cervical Tenderpoints
Location:
Usually slightly anterior to or on the most lateral aspect of the lateral masses. [1 p.758]
Treatment position:
Most are treated in flexion with sidebending away and rotating the patient's head away from the side of the tenderpoint. [32 p.156]

Posterior Cervical Tenderpoints
Location:
Usually on the occiput or at the tip of the correstponding spinous process or on the lateral sides of the corresponding spinous process. [32 p.161, 1 p.758]
Treatment Position:
Most are treated with extension, sidebending away (slightly), and rotate away. [32 p.161]

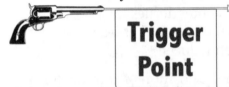

> **MEMORY TOOL:**
> SARA - Sidebend Away Rotate Away = treatment position for most anterior and posterior cervical tenderpoints.

B. Thoracic Spine

Anterior Thoracic Tenderpoints
Location: [1 p.758, 32 p.167]
AT1-AT6: Located at the midline of the sternum at the attachment of the corresponding ribs.
AT7-AT11: Located in the rectus abdominus muscle about one inch lateral to the midline on the right or left.
AT12: Anterior superior surface of the iliac crest at the midaxillary line.
Treatment Position:
Flex, sidebend toward and rotate away.

Posterior Thoracic Tenderpoints
Location:
PT1-PT12: Located on either side of the corresponding spinous process or on the transverse process. [1 p.758, 32 p.173]
Treatment Position
Extend and sidebend away (rotation away if tenderpoint is on the spinous process, rotate toward if tenderpoint on transverse process) [32 p.173]

C. __Ribs__

Anterior tenderpoints are associated with depressed ribs (now presumed to be similar to an exhalation dysfunction). Posterior tenderpoints are associated with elevated ribs (inhalation dysfunction).[1 p.759, 32 p.180,183, 22 p.379]

Jones recommends maintaining rib treatment positions for 120 seconds to allow the patient extra time to relax.[1 p.755]

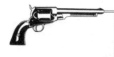

Trigger Point

Anterior rib tenderpoints associated with Exhalation dysfunctions

Posterior rib tenderpoints associated with Inhalation dysfunctions

__Anterior Rib Tenderpoints__

Location: [32 p.179]

Rib 1 (AR1): Below the clavicle on the first condrosternal junction.

Rib 2(AR2): On rib 2 at the mid-clavicular line

Ribs 3-10 (AR3-10): Located along the anterior axillary line on the corresponding rib.

Treatment Position: [32 p.179]

Flexion, sidebend and rotate towards.

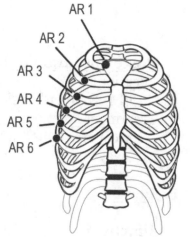

Fig. 14.1: *Anterior rib tenderpoints*

__Posterior Rib Tenderpoints__

Location: [32 p.182]

Rib 1 (PR1): On rib one lateral to the costotransverse articulation

Rib 2-10 (PR2-10):The angle of the corresponding rib.

Treatment Position: [32 p. 182, 44 p.82, 33 p.66]

Rib 1: slight extension, sidebend away rotate toward

Rib2-10: minimal flexion, sidebend away and rotate away.

D. Lumbar Spine
Anterior Lumbar Tenderpoints
Location: [32 p.185]

> L1 (AL1): Medial to the ASIS.
> L2-L4 (AL2-4): On the AIIS.
> L5 (AL5): One cm lateral to the pubic symphysis on the superior ramus.

Treatment Position:

> Most are treated with the patient supine, knees and hips flexed. Sidebending is added by moving the ankles right or left. Rotation is added by pulling the knees right or left.

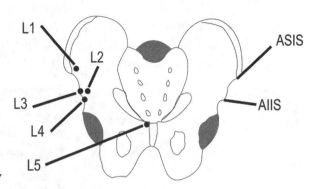

Fig. 14.2: *Anterior lumbar tenderpoints*

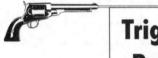

Trigger Point

The anterior tenderpoint for L5 is located one cm lateral to the pubic symphysis on the superior ramus.

Posterior Lumbar Tenderpoints
Location: [32 p.195]

> PL1-5: On either side of the spinous process or on the transverse process.

Treatment Position:

> Most are treated with the patient prone, extended and sidebent and rotated away

E. Pelvis

Iliacus:
Location:

> Approximately 7 cm medial to the ASIS.

Treatment Position:

> Patient supine with the hip flexed and externally rotated.

Piriformis
Location: [1 p.760]

> Usually in the piriformis muscle 7 cm medial to and slightly cephalad to the greater trochanter.

Treatment position: [1 p.760]

> Pt prone. Hip and knee flexed. Thigh abducted and externally rotated.

III. Facilitated Positional Release (FPR)

A. Definition

A system of indirect myofascial release treatment developed by Stanley Schiowitz, DO. The component region of the body is placed into a neutral position, diminishing tissue and joint tension in all planes. An activating force (compression or torsion) is added. [1 p.1097] It is easily applied, nontraumatic, and only takes 3-4 seconds to induce a release.

General steps for facilitated positional release:
1. Place spine in neutral position
2. Apply facilitatiing force
3. Place dysfunctional tissue in shortened relaxed position
4. Hold for 3-4 seconds
5. Reevaluate

FPR Technique can be used to treat:
1. Superficial muscles
2. Deep intervertebral muscles to influence vertebral motion

Typical FPR Procedure

Superficial Muscle Treatment
1. With the patient in a neutral position, the physician first straightens the AP curvature of the spine (decreasing the kyphosis or lordosis).
2. The physician then applies the facilitating force (compression or torsion, or both).
3. The physician then shortens the muscle to be treated.
4. The position is held for 3 to 4 seconds.
5. The physician releases the position and reevaluates the dysfunction.

Deep intervertebral muscle treatment (Intervertebral motion treatment)

Diagnosis C5 ES_RR_R:
1. The patient is supine, with his/her head beyond the end of the table, resting in a pillow in the physician's lap.
2. With the patient in a neutral position, straighten the cervical lordosis by flexing the head slightly.
3. The physician then applies the facilitating force (compression or torsion, or both).
4. The physician will then place C5 in ES_RR_R using the head as a lever.
5. The position is held for 3 to 4 seconds.
6. The physician releases the position and reevaluates the dysfunction.

Chapter 14 Review Questions

1. A soccer player presents with hip pain after playing in a tournament. Structural examination reveals a tenderpoint for the iliacus muscle. A small tense area of edema would be best appreciated

    A. 1 cm lateral to the ASIS
    B. 3 cm medial to the ASIS
    C. 5 cm lateral to the ASIS
    D. 7 cm medial to the ASIS
    E. over the ASIS

2. A 58-year-old male presents with left upper chest pain of 2 months duration. Structural examination reveals a tenderpoint on rib 2. The anterior counterstrain point for the affected area is located at the

    A. anterior axillary line
    B. mid-clavicular line
    C. most lateral aspect of the rib
    D. posterior axillary line
    E. sternal junction

3. A 40-year-old male presents with chronic radicular back pain radiating down the right leg. Physical examination reveals tenderness of the piriformis muscle. During the counterstrain technique with the patient prone, which of the following motions are introduced during the course of the procedure?

    A. abduction of the hip and external rotation of the thigh
    B. abduction of the hip and internal rotation of the thigh
    C. abduction of the hip, hip flexion, and traction through the femur
    D. adduction of the hip and internal rotation of the thigh
    E. adduction of the hip, hip extension, and external rotation of the thigh

4. A young female presents with chronic neck pain. She reports it is worst when she is driving and trying to look over her shoulder. Range of motion testing is pertinent for reduced active and passive cervical rotation to the left. Exam demonstrates a painful tenderpoint on the C5 lateral mass. The proper treatment position of this tenderpoint involves

    A. flexion, sidebending, and rotation towards the point
    B. pure rotation away from the point
    C. flexion, sidebending and rotation away from the point
    D. rotation towards the point, sidebending away

E. sidebending towards the point, rotation away

5. A 70-year-old male presents male presents with neck pain after golfing. He points to a specific location at the tip of the spinous process as the origin of his pain. When treating these types of cervical tenderpoints using counterstrain, the provider should

    A. flex the neck until maximal comfort is obtained at the tenderpoint
    B. have the patient move the cervical spine to neutral position after treatment
    C. hold the treatment position for 120 seconds
    D. locate the tenderpoints along the anterolateral tips of the lateral masses of the cervical vertebrae
    E. slowly extend the head and cervical spine down to the tenderpoint

6. When utilizing facilitated positional release to a superficial muscle, which is performed first?

    A. application of compression
    B. application of traction
    C. fine tuning the position
    D. shortening of the hypertonic muscle
    E. straightening the AP curves

7. A 55-year-old presents with neck pain after a motor vehicle accident. Examination reveals a more prominent left transverse process of C4 in the extended position, and thus the patient is setup for cervical facilitated positional release. The facilitating force for this technique is

    A. compression
    B. cranial balancing
    C. extension
    D. rotation
    E. sidebending

Questions 8-11 refer to the following:

An elderly male presents with chronic back pain after a remote motor vehicle accident. He takes over the counter analgesics which is effective enough for him to complete his activities of daily living. Osteopathic manipulative treatment is employed using the counterstrain technique due to his age and the patient is setup into the appropriate treatment position.

8. When fine tuning position for a counterstrain technique, what is the minimum acceptable reduction of pain?

    A. 30%
    B. 60%
    C. 70%
    D. 85%
    E. 95%

9. When performing counterstrain technique, you should

    A. engage the anatomic barrier
    B. engage the restrictive barrier
    C. find the balance point where equal forces exists across the joint in all directions
    D. monitor the tender point with your finger, but without excess digital pressure
    E. squeeze the tissue firmly with rotatory movement until tissue texture changes resolve

10. In counterstrain technique, the role of the finger over the tenderpoint is to

    A. apply about 10 kg of pressure
    B. inhibitory and rotatory pressure
    C. monitor for change
    D. provide a fulcrum for patient positioning
    E. stimulate the tenderpoint

11. The location of the tenderpoint is most likely

    A. along the course of a sensory nerve
    B. in the belly or tendon of the shortened muscle
    C. in the antagonist to the shortened muscle
    D. in the contralateral muscle or tendon
    E. in the mid-coronal plane

Questions 12-13 refer to the following:
    A patient presents with back pain and is diagnosed with somatic dysfunction of T10 and L5.

12. Which of the following represents the corresponding location for the anterior thoracic tenderpoint for this segment?

    A. approximately 1 inch lateral and ½ inch inferior to umbilicus bilaterally
    B. approximately 1 ½ inches inferior to the umbilicus
    C. approximately 2 inches inferior to the sternal notch in the midline
    D. at the sternal notch
    E. on the iliac crest in the mid-axillary line bilaterally

13. The anterior lumbar tenderpoint for L5 is located at

    A. directly over the pubic symphysis
    B. lateral to the ASIS
    C. medial to the ASIS
    D. medial to the AIIS
    E. over the pubic ramus 1cm from the symphysis

Explanations

1. Answer: **D**

    The iliacus is a flat triangular muscle that arises from the iliac fossa and inserts on the lesser trochanter to flex the hip. The location of the tenderpoint associated with dysfunction of the iliacus is approximately 7 cm medial to the ASIS. Treatment involves flexion and external rotation of the hip with the patient supine.

2. Answer: **B**

    The anterior rib tenderpoint for rib 2 is located at the mid-clavicular line. Treatment involves flexion with sidebending and rotation towards the somatic dysfunction.

3. Answer: **A**

    The piriformis tenderpoint is usually found 7cm medial to and slightly cephalad to the greater trochanter. The treatment position involves the patient in the prone position with the knee and hip flexed. The thigh is then abducted and hip externally rotated.

4. Answer: **C**

    Anterior cervial tenderpoints are usually located slightly anterior to or on the most lateral aspect of the lateral masses. [1 p.758] Treatment using counterstrain involves shortening the affected muscle or tendon which is best done with flexion, sidebending and rotating from the tenderpoint.   Of note, the tenderpoint associated with C1 (atlas) is treated with primarily rotation away from the tenderpoint (very little flexion and sidebending away).

5. Answer: **E**

    Posterior cervical tenderpoints are found at the tip or lateral sides of the corresponding spinous process. They are usually treated in the extended position with the head slightly sidebent away and rotated away from the tenderpoint. First the tenderpoint is located, the tenderness scale is assessed, and then the patient is placed into a position of optimal comfort. After 90 seconds the physician slowly returns the neck to the neutral position and re-evaluates the tenderpoint.

6. Answer: **E**

Typical superficial muscle treatment first involves straightening the anterior-posterior (AP) curvature such as flattening a thoracic kyphosis or lumbar lordosis. Then the facilitating force is applied and muscle belly shortened. The treatment position is held for 3-4 seconds and then released.

7. Answer: **A**

The patient's C4 is extended, rotated left, sidebent left (C4 ERSL). After the AP curve is flattened then a facilitating force is applied and maintained, followed by decreasing the length of the involved muscle and/or further positioning of the somatic dysfunction into all three planes of relative freedom. The facilitating force is usually compression and/or torsion.

8. Answer: **C**

Counterstrain is a passive indirect technique in which the tissue being treated is positioned away from the restrictive barrier. It is well tolerated in the elderly. During treatment you should maintain light contact to monitor the tenderpoint and make gross movements in order to shortened the muscle being treated. Then, fine tune the involved planes of movement with small degrees of movement until at least 70% of the tenderness has been reduced.

9. Answer: **D**

Please refer to the explanation for item number 8.

10. Answer: **C**

Please refer to the explanation for item number 8.

11. Answer: **B**

Counterstrain tenderpoints are typically located near bony attachments of tendons, ligaments, or in the belly of some muscles.

12. Answer: **A**

The anterior thoracic tenderpoint for T7-T11 is in the rectus abdominus muscle about one inch lateral to the midline on the right or left. The corresponding posterior tenderpoint would be found at the spinous process or on the transverse process.

13. Answer: **E**

The anterior lumbar tenderpoint for L5 is found 1 cm lateral to the pubic symphysis on the superior ramus. The corresponding posterior tenderpoint would be found at the spinous process or on the transverse process.

Muscle Energy 15

I. Definition

Muscle energy is a form of OMT in which the patient actively uses his muscles on request, "from a precisely controlled position in a specific direction, against a distinctly executed counterforce." [1 p.1098]

II. Principles of Muscle Energy Treatment

Muscle energy can be performed as an active direct or active indirect technique (see Chapter 1, The Basics for further description of these types of treatments).

NOTE: Most forms of muscle energy treatment are direct. Indirect is rarely used.

III. Types of Muscle Energy

1. Postisometric relaxation (direct technique): The physician, after correct diagnosis of the somatic dysfunction, reverses all components in all planes and engages the restrictive barrier.

   The physician then instructs the patient to contract equally against the offered counterforce by the physician. This isometric contraction, where the distance between the origin and the insertion of the muscle remains the same as the muscle contracts, will stretch the internal connective tissues.

   The Golgi tendon organs sense this change in tension in the muscle tendons and causes a reflex relaxation of the agonist muscle fibers.[61 p.685] Therefore, by reflex relaxation of the agonist muscle, the physician is then able to passively stretch the patient in all planes of motion to the new restrictive barrier.

For example, if the biceps muscle is in spasm, extend the elbow fully to the restrictive barrier, flex the biceps against resistance for 3-5 seconds, then relax. Extend the elbow to the new restrictive barrier, then repeat. The force of muscle contraction should be approximately 10-20lbs.[1 p. 685] It is not a competition to see who is stronger.

Since the agonist muscle is most likely the dysfunctional muscle, this type of muscle energy is most useful in *subacute or chronic conditions* where muscle shortening and fibrosis is present, rather than acute conditions.[32 p.247]

2. Reciprocal inhibition: Another muscle energy technique that utilizes the reflex mechanism of reciprocal inhibition when antagonistic muscles are contracted.

    By contracting the antagonistic muscle, signals are transmitted to the spinal cord and through the reciprocal inhibition reflex arc. The agonist muscle is then forced to relax. This technique is most useful in *acute conditions*, since gentle contraction of the antagonist muscle will put little strain on the dysfunctional agonist. The amount of muscle contraction is minimal (think ounces - not pounds).[1 p.685]

    Reciprocal inhibition can be done directly[7 p.311] **or indirectly.**[7 p.680]

    a. Reciprocal inhibition - direct technique
        If the biceps muscle is in spasm, extend the elbow fully to the restrictive barrier, then have the patient contract their triceps against resistance. This isometric force through reciprocal inhibition allows the biceps muscle to relax and return to a normal resting state.

    b. Reciprocal inhibition - indirect technique (rare)
        If the biceps muscle is in spasm, fully flex the elbow (away from the restrictive barrier), then have the patient contract their triceps against resistance. This isometric force through reciprocal inhibition allows the biceps muscle to relax and return to a normal resting state.

3. Joint mobilization using muscle force: This type of muscle energy restores normal range of motion of a joint using muscle contraction.[1 p.685] The force of muscle contraction should be what can be comfortably resisted by the physician (30 - 50lbs). For example, contracting the hip flexors helps pull the innominate anterior in a posterior innominate dysfunction.

4. Oculocephalogyric reflex: This type of muscle energy uses extraocular muscle contraction to reflexively effect the cervical and truncal musculature.[1 p.883] The patient can be asked to look toward the restriction (reciprocal inhibition effect) or away from the restriction (postisometric effect).[32 p.248] This technique is useful for severe acute upper thoracic and cervical conditions.

5. <u>Respiratory assistance</u>: This type of muscle energy uses the patient's voluntary respiratory motion to restore normal motion.[1 p.685] Most inhalation rib dysfunctions are treated in this fashion.

6. <u>Crossed extensor reflex</u>: This form of muscle energy uses the crossed extensor reflex to achieve muscle relaxation. It is typically used in extremities that are so severely injured or not accessable that direct manipulation is impossible. For example, contraction of the right biceps produces relaxation of the left biceps and contraction of the left triceps. The amount of muscle contraction is minimal, (think ounces - not pounds).[1 p.685]

Table 15.1

Types of Muscle Energy	Indications	Force used
Postisometric relaxation	Subacute or Chronic	10 - 20 lbs
Recriprocal inhibition	Acute	Ounces
Joint mobilization using muscle force	Restore motion in joint dysfunction	30 - 50 lbs
Oculocephalogyric reflex	Very severe acute cervical and upper thoracic conditions	Very gentle
Respiratory assistance	Commonly used in rib inhalation dysfunctions	Exaggerated respiration
Crossed extensor reflex	When effected extremity is unmanipulatable or inaccessable	Ounces

V. <u>Typical Muscle Energy Treatment Sequence</u>

1. The physician positions the bone or joint so the muscle group will engage the restrictive barrier (direct treatment) in all planes of motion.
2. The operator instructs the patient to reverse direction in one or all planes of motion.
3. The patient contracts the appropriate muscle(s) or muscle group with the objective of moving the body part through a complete range of motion.
4. The physician maintains an appropriate counterforce so that the contraction is perceived at the critical articulation or area for 3-5 seconds.
5. The physician then instructs the patient to relax and the physician also relaxes. Then during the post-isometric relaxation phase, the physician takes up the slack, allowing it to be passively lengthened. Increased range of motion is noted by the physician.
6. Steps 1-5 are repeated for 3-5 times until the best possible increase in motion is obtained.

VI. <u>Indications</u>

1. Lengthen shortened muscles/stretch or improve elasticity in fibrotic muscles
2. Mobilize restricted joints and improve range of motion

VII. <u>Contraindications</u>

1. Moderate to severe muscle strains
2. Severe osteoporosis
3. Severe illness (postsurgical or ICU patients)
4. Fracture/dislocation or severe joint instabilty at treatment site

VIII. <u>Muscle Energy Techniques</u>

<u>Cervical Spine</u>
Positional Diagnosis: OA ES_LR_R
Treatment Position: supine

1. With the distal pad of one finger, monitor the OA joint, engage the restrictive barrier in all three planes by sidebending right, rotating left and flexing the patient's head until tension is felt under your monitoring finger. This is called localization. Direct the patient to use a small amount of force to straighten their head while you exert an equal amount of counterforce.
2. Maintain the forces for 3-5 seconds, repeat 3-5 times, each time re-engaging the new restrictive barrier.
3. Recheck for symmetry of motion.

Positional Diagnosis: AA R_R
Treatment Position: supine

1. Cradle the occiput in your hands and flex the patient's cervical spine 45°, locking out all the facets below the AA joint.
2. Rotate the atlas to the left to the point of initial resistance.
3. Direct the patient to gently rotate their head to the right. Apply an equal counterforce through your fingers and hands.
4. Maintain the forces for 3-5 seconds, repeat 3-5 times, each time re-engaging the new restrictive barrier.
5. Recheck for symmetry of motion.

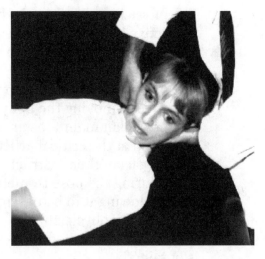

Fig. 15.1: Treatment of AA R_R

Typical Cervicals (C2-C7)
Positional Diagnosis: C3 ER_RS_R

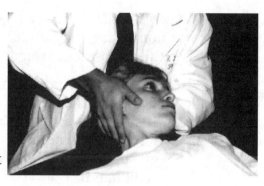

1. With the distal pad of one finger on the articular pillar of the dysfunctional segment, engage the restrictive barrier by reversing the somatic dysfunction in all three planes of motion until motion is felt under your monitoring finger. Remember that *rotation and sidebending components are to the same side.*

Fig. 15.2: *Treatment of C3 ER_RS_R*

2. Direct the patient to gently straighten their head while you apply an equal counterforce.
3. Repeat steps 4-5 in the above example.

Thoracic Spine
Upper Thoracic Spine (T1-T4)
Positional Diagnosis: T3 ES_LR_L
Treatment Position: seated

1. In the upper thoracic spine the physician will use the head and neck as lever to induce motion at the dysfunctional segment.

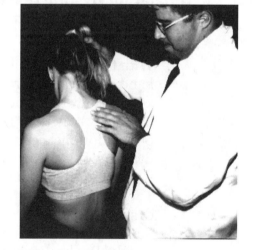

2. With one hand monitor the posterior transverse process of T3. Engage the restrictive barrier by flexing, rotating and sidebending right until motion is felt under your monitoring finger.
3. Direct the patient to use a small amount of force to straighten their head while you exert an equal amount of counterforce.
4. Maintain the forces for 3-5 seconds, have the patient relax, the physician relaxes, and re-engage the new restrictive barrier.

Fig. 15.3: *Treatment of T3 ES_LR_L*

5. Repeat step four 3-5 times and then recheck for increased symmetry.

Lower Thoracic Spine (T5-T12)
Positional Diagnosis: T7 ER_LS_L
Treatment Position: Seated

1. Use your left hand to monitor the posterior transverse process of T7.
2. Instruct the patient to place their left hand behind their neck, and to grasp their left elbow with their right hand.
3. Reach across the patient's chest with your right arm, sidebending and rotating T7 to the right until motion is felt under your monitoring finger.
4. Direct the patient to use a small amount of force to straighten his body while you exert an equal amount of counterforce.
5. Repeat step four 3-5 times and then recheck for increased symmetry.

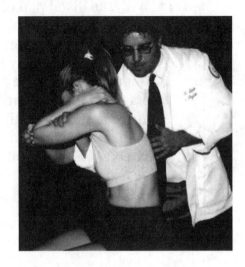

Fig. 15.4: Treatment of T7 ER_LS_L

Ribs
Inhalation Dysfunctions (rib held up)
Treatment Position: supine
Key Rib: Lowest in group

1. With the patient supine, place one hand on the anterior aspect of the key rib. Flex the patient for pump handle dysfunctions (sidebend the patient for bucket handle dysfunctions) down so that tension is taken off the dysfunctional rib
2. The physician palpates the dysfuncitonal rib.
3. Patient inhales, then exhales deeply. For bucket handle dysfunctions, patient is instructed to reach for their knee on the affected side.

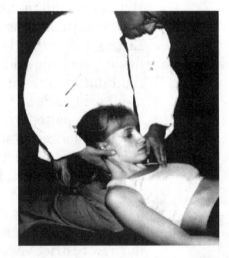

Fig. 15.5: Treatment of a Pump-handle dysfunction of Rib 4

4. The patient is instructed to hold their breath at end-expiratory phase for 3-5 seconds. During this time, the physician adjusts flexion/sidebending to the new restrictive barrier. Physician follows rib shaft into exhalation with his hand during the expiratory phase.
5. On inhalation, the physician resists inhalation motion of the rib.
6. Repeat steps 3-5 a total of 3-5 times. Retest for symmetry of motion.

Exhalation Dysfunctions (rib held down)

NOTE: There are many different methods used when treating exhalation dysfunctions. Techniques differ slightly. The important concept of these rib treatments is to keep in mind which muscle is being used to correct the dysfunction. This is summarized in table 15.2

Treatment Position: Supine

Key Rib: Top Rib in Group

1. The patient is instructed to place the forearm on the affected side across his forehead with the palm up.

2. The physician grasps the key rib posteriorly at the rib angle.

3. The patient is instructed to inhale deeply while the physician applies an inferior traction on the rib angle.

4. The patient is instructed to hold his breath at full inhalation while performing one of the following isometric contractions for 3-5 seconds:
   a. Rib 1-2:
      Patient turns head 30 degrees away from dysfunctional side and lifts head toward ceiling.
   b. Ribs 3-5:
      Patient pushes elbow of affected side toward the opposite ASIS.
   c. Ribs 6-8:
      Push arm anterior.
   d. Ribs 9-10:
      Patient adducts arm.

5. Repeat step 4 a total of 3-5 times and then retest.

a 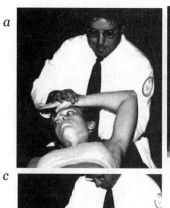 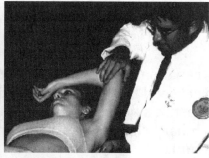 b

c 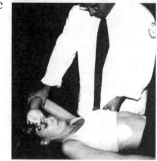 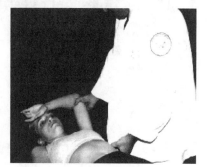 d

Figures 15.6:

a: Treatment of exhalation dysfunction of Rib 1-2 on the left.

b: Treatment of exhalation dysfunction Ribs 3-5 on the left.

c: Treatment of exhalation dysfunction of Ribs 6-8 on the left.

d: Treatment of exhalation dysfunction of Ribs 9-10 on the left.

Table 15.2 [64 p.275-85]

Ribs	Muscles
Rib 1	Anterior and Middle Scalenes
Rib 2	Posterior Scalene
Ribs 3-5	Pectoralis Minor
Ribs 6-8	Serratus Anterior
Ribs 9-10	Latissimus Dorsi
Rib 11-12	Quadratus Lumborum

Lumbar Spine: Lumbar seated technique
Positional Diagnosis: $L3E_RS_R$
Same steps as the lower thoracic spine.

Sacrum:
Unilateral Sacral Flexion
Positional Diagnosis: Right USF
Treatment Position: prone

1. Place your left hypothenar eminence on the patient's right ILA.
2. Ask the patient to inhale and hold their breath, while you push anteriorly on the ILA. Hold for 3-5 seconds.
3. Direct the patient to exhale while you resist any posterior inferior movement of the sacrum.
4. Repeat steps two and three 3-5 times and retest.

Unilateral Sacral Extension
Positional Diagnosis: Right USE
Treatment Position: prone

1. Place your left hypothenar eminence on the patient's right sacral sulcus.
2. Ask the patient to exhale and hold their breath, while you push anterior and caudad on the superior sulcus. Hold for 3-5 seconds.
3. Direct the patient to inhale while you resist any anterior superior movement of the sacrum.
4. Repeat steps two and three 3-5 times and retest.

Sacral Torsions:

Positional Diagnosis: Left on Left (forward sacral torsion)

Treatment Position: left lateral lims position (lying on left side with face down)

1. Patient lies on their left side (_axis side down_) with their torso rotated so that they are face down.
2. Flex patient's hips until motion is felt at the lumbosacral junction.
3. Drop the patient's legs off the table to induce left sidebending and engage a left sacral oblique axis.
4. Ask the patient to lift their legs toward the ceiling against your equal counterforce for 3-5 seconds. Monitor with other hand the right superior pole for posterior movement.
5. Repeat for 3-5 times and then retest for symmetry.

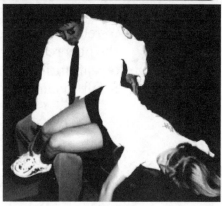

MEMORY TOOL:

Forward sacral torsion patient lies **F**ace down.

Fig. 15.7: Treatment of a Left on Left Forward Sacral Torsion

Positional Diagnosis: Right on Left (backward sacral torsion)

Treatment Position: left lateral recumbent with face up

1. Patient lies on theri left side (axis side down) with their torso rotated so that they is face up.
2. Grasp patient's left arm and pull through to rotate their torso to the right. Flex patient's hips until motion is felt at the lumbosacral junction.
3. Drop the patient's legs off the table to induce left sidebending and engage a left sacral oblique axis.
4. Ask the patient to lift their legs toward the ceiling against your equal counterforce for 3-5 seconds. Monitor with other hand the right superior pole for anterior movement.
5. Repeat for 3-5 times, each time re-engaging the new restrictive barrier, and retest for symmetry of motion.

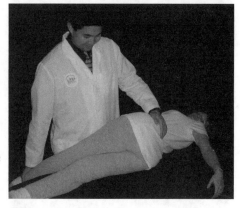

MEMORY TOOL:

Backward sacral torsion patient lies on their **B**ack.

Fig. 15.8: Treatment of a Right on Left, Backward Sacral Torsion.

Innominates:

Positional Diagnosis: right innominate anterior
Treatment Position: supine

1. Flex patient's right hip and knee until resistance is felt.
2. Instruct patient to extend their hip against your counterforce for 3-5 seconds.
3. Wait a few seconds for the tissues to relax, then take up the slack to the new restrictive barrier.
4. Repeat until no restrictive barrier is felt (usually 3-5 times).

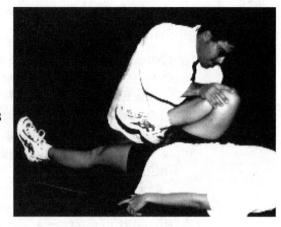

Fig. 15.9: Treatment of a Right Innominate Anterior.

Positional Diagnosis: right innominate posterior
Treatment Position: supine

1. Drop the patient's right leg off the table until resistance is felt. Stabilize the patient's left ASIS with your right hand.
2. Instruct patient to flex his their against your counterforce for 3-5 seconds.
3. Repeat steps 3 and 4.

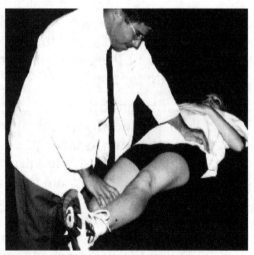

Fig. 15.10: Treatment of a Right Innominate Posterior.

Pubic Shears:

Positional Diagnosis: right superior pubic shear
Treatment Position: supine

1. Drop the patient's right leg off the table and abduct until resistance is felt. Stabilize the patient's left ASIS with your right hand.
2. Instruct patient to bring their right knee to their left ASIS (flexion and adduction) against your counterforce for 3-5 seconds.
3. Repeat steps 3 and 4.

Positional Diagnosis: right inferior pubic shear
Treatment Position: supine

1. Flex and abduct patient's right hip and knee and until resistance is felt. Stabilize the patient's left ASIS with your right hand.
2. Instruct patient to push thieir right knee to his their foot (extension and adduction) against your counterforce for 3-5 seconds.
3. Repeat steps 3-4.

Upper Extremities:

Positional Diagnosis: Right forearm has restriction of supination (radial head posterior).
Treatment Position: seated

1. Place your right hand at the distal end of the patient's right forearm and supinate it to initial resistance as you monitor with the other thumb at the radial head.
2. Direct the patient to pronate the right forearm against equal resistance supplied through your right hand.
3. Maintain the forces long enough to sense the patient's contractile force at the localized segment or area (usually 3-5 seconds).
4. Both the patient and physician relax their forces, and the physician takes up the slack to the new point of initial resistance.
5. Repeat for 3-5 times and then recheck findings.

Positional Diagnosis: Right forearm has restriction of pronation (radial head anterior).
Treatment Position: seated

1. Support the patient's right elbow with your left hand.
2. Place your right hand at the distal end of the patient's right forearm and pronate it to initial resistance.
3. Direct the patient to supinate the right forearm against an equal counterforce supplied through your right hand.
4. Maintain the force for 3-5 seconds, then both the physician and the patient relaxes. The physician then re-engages the new restrictive barrier. Repeat for 3-5 times and then recheck findings.

Lower Extremities

<u>NOTE</u>: There are many different methods used when correcting fibular head dysfunctions. Techniques differ slightly. The following techniques have been described by Fred Mitchell, DO. [45]

Positional Diagnosis: Right fibular head anterior [45 p.550]
Treatment Position: prone

1. With the patient in the prone position and the knee flexed, place your right hand on the lateral side of the patient's foot, cupping the ankle.
2. Plantarflex and invert the patient's foot to initial resistance.
3. Externally rotate the tibia.
4. Direct the patient to dorsiflex against your isometric counterforce for 3-5 seconds.
5. Relax forces, plantar-flex, invert and externally rotate the tibia to the new barrier. Repeat steps 1-4.

Positional Diagnosis: Right fibular head posterior [45 p.550]
Treatment Position: prone

1. With the patient in the prone position and the knee flexed, place your right hand on the lateral side of the patient's foot, cupping the ankle.
2. Plantar-flex and invert the patient's foot to initial resistance.
3. Internally rotate the tibia
4. Direct the patient to dorsiflex against your isometric counterforce for 3-5 seconds.
5. Relax forces, plantarflex, invert and internally rotate the tibia to the new barrier. Repeat steps 1-4.

Chapter 15 Review Questions

1. Which of the following is a necessary component for any successful muscle energy treatment?

    A. direct treatment to the pathologic barrier
    B. holding the position for 90 seconds
    C. patient assistance
    D. post-isometric relaxation
    E. reciprocal inhibition

2. An 18-year-old male presents with right-sided chest pain after a coughing fit. Structural examination reveals an inhaled rib on the right side at the Angle of Louis. Which of the following muscles help elevate this rib with forced inhalation?

    A. anterior scalene
    B. middle scalene
    C. pectoralis minor
    D. posterior scalene
    E. sternocleidomastoid

3. A 15-year-old male presents with chest pain after a football injury. The pain is worse with inhalation. Physical examination reveals the lungs are clear to auscultation and the ribs are without point tenderness. Structural examination reveals the following:

    • Prominence of the anterosuperior and posteroinferior surfaces of rib 10 on the right
    • Decreased excursion of rib 10 on the right during inhalation

    Plain film radiography is negative for fracture. Which muscle is used to treat this dysfunction when using a muscle energy technique?

    A. iliocostalis
    B. latissimus dorsi
    C. serratus anterior
    D. serratus posterior
    E. quadratus lumborum

4. In which patient would muscle energy techniques be CONTRAINDICATED?

    A. 6-year-old healthy child
    B. 23-year-old paraplegic
    C. 38-year-old female immediately post-MI
    D. 45-year-old male with GERD
    E. 76-year-old healthy man

5. A 45-year-old truck driver presents with chronic low back pain that radiates down the left leg. It seemed to improve after he stopped putting his wallet on his back left side. Structural examination reveals a hypertonic piriformis on the left and the patient is placed into position using muscle energy. While in this position the patient's hip is

    A. abducted
    B. adducted
    C. externally rotated
    D. internally rotated
    E. laterally translated

6. A 30-year-old male presents with thoracic back pain described with an aching quality. Examination reveals that T8 rotates and sidebends more freely to the left. These movements appear to improve with extension rather than flexion. The patient is consented for osteopathic manipulation using muscle energy and put into the treatment position. The patient's position just prior to isometric contraction will be

    A. extended, rotated left, sidebent left with active sidebending to the right
    B. extended, rotated right, sidebent right with active sidebending to the right
    C. flexed, rotated left, sidebent left with active sidebending to the left
    D. flexed, rotated right, sidebent right with active sidebending to the left
    E. flexed, rotated right, sidebent right with active sidebending to the right

7. 20-year-old female presents for a general maintenance examination without complaints. A comprehensive musculoskeletal examination is unremarkable. Structural examination is reveals minor tissue texture changes in the cervical and thoracic regions and the practitioner sets up the patient for muscle energy technique. Which joint is treated by the use of rotational force only?

    A. OA
    B. AA
    C. C3
    D. T2
    E. posterior radial head

8. A patient with low back pain is placed in position for osteopathic manipulation using muscle energy. The physician finds the restrictive barrier and then asks the patient to contract a muscle against resistance for

    A. 1-2 seconds
    B. 3-5 seconds
    C. 90 seconds
    D. 120 seconds
    E. 1-2 minutes

A 24-year-old female presents with pelvic pain of 4 months' duration. Structural examination reveals the right ASIS is more superior, there are tissue texture changes at the right sacral sulcus, and also mild tenderness in the inguinal region. Standing flexion test is positive on the right.

9. When positioning the patient to treat the most likely diagnosis using muscle energy, the patient is

    A. prone with the right thigh lifted off the table
    B. prone with the right thigh abducted and dropped off the table
    C. supine with both feet placed on the table and the right foot slightly inferior to the left
    D. supine with the right thigh flexed to 120 degrees
    E. supine with the right thigh lowered off the table

10. The patient is asked to contract the

    A. left hamstring
    B. left hip flexors
    C. right erector spinae muscles
    D. right hamstring
    E. right hip flexors

Questions 11-12 refer to the following:

A 30-year-old male presents for follow-up for allergic rhinitis. He complains that when he sneezes frequently and feels some discomfort in his upper chest. While evaluating the pump handle mechanics of his respiratory cycle, you notice rib 2 is restricted with inhalation. The patient is consented for muscle energy using a post-isometric relaxation technique.

11. The patient is placed in position for treatment using muscle energy, during which the

    A. arm is adducted isometrically from a position of 90 degrees of abduction
    B. patient pushes his head into extension
    C. patient pushes his head into flexion with his forearm flexed on his forehead
    D. pectoralis minor muscle is isolated
    E. serratus anterior is utilized

12. Which of the following describes the standard steps of this technique?

    A. engage the barrier, patient contracts against the physician's counterforce for 3-5 seconds, engage the new barrier, repeat 3 times

    B. engage the barrier, patient contracts against the physician's counterforce for 3-5 seconds, relax 1-2 seconds, engage the new barrier, repeat 3 times

    C. engage the barrier, thrust and hold for 3-5 seconds, relax 1-2 seconds, repeat 3 times

    D. take the patient away from the barrier, the patient contracts against the physician's counterforce for 3-5 seconds, relax 1-2 seconds, repeat 3 times

    E. take the patient away from the barrier, thrust and hold for 3-5 seconds, relax 1-2 seconds, repeat 3 times

Explanations

1. Answer: **C**

   Muscle energy requires patient-mediate muscle activation in order to work. After the muscle is put into the treatment position the patient is requested to engage in isometric muscle contraction which is not possible without patient assistance.

2. Answer: **D**

   The angle of Louis is the anatomic landmark for the sternal angle and attaches to the 2nd rib. The posterior scalene attaches to the second rib and can help to elevate this exhaled rib with forced inhalation. Refer to the Chapter 3 Thorax and Ribcage for more information on treatment of rib dysfunctions.

3. Answer: **B**

   The patient has an exhalation dysfunction of rib 10 which is best treated when activating the latissimus dorsi muscle. Please refer to Table 15.2 for more information.

4. Answer: **C**

   There are relatively few absolute contraindications for osteopathic manipulation. For muscle energy specifically, any acute or medically unstable patient who should otherwise be resting should avoid treatment. For example, someone who has a DVT, fracture, trauma, was recently recovering from surgery or an acute MI should not be excessively mobilizes until their condition stabilizes.

5. Answer: **D**

   The treatment position involves the patient in a prone position with the knee flexed and hip internally rotated until the initial resistance is palpated. The practicioner's hand is placed on the medial aspect of the ankle and the patient is asked to externally rotate into the provider's hand for 3-5 seconds.

6. Answer: **D**

The patient has somatic dysfunction with a T8 that is extended, rotated and sidebent left (T8 ERS$_L$). Recall that somatic dysfunction is named for the freedom of motion. T8 rotates and sidebends more freely to the left, so it is named as rotated/sidebent left. Since the dysfunctions with extension, it is named as extended. Lower thoracic dysfunctions are best treated in the seated position while moving all planes into the restrictive barrier. For this patient it would be flexion with rotation and sidebending to the right. The patient's movement involves sidebending back to the left as the corrective force.

7. Answer: **B**

The atlas rests on the axis to create the atlantoaxial (AA) joint which accounts for at least 50% of cervical rotation. This joint primarily rotates and therefore the treatment position only involves rotation.

8. Answer: **B**

Muscle energy involves patient participation wherein the agonist muscle is contracted against resistance for 3-5 seconds.

9. Answer: **E**

The patient has a right posterior innominate rotation. Treatment is in the supine position with the leg dropped off of the side of the table until resistance is appreciated. The patient is then instructed to flex the hip against a counterforce for 3-5 seconds.

10. Answer: **E**

See explanation for Question 9.

11. Answer: **C**

This patient has an exhalation dysfunction due to freer motion during exhalation with restriction during inhalation. Muscle energy for ribs involves the patient in the supine position with the forearm on the affected side across the forehead and the physician holding the rib posteriorly on the rib angle, applying traction upon inhalation. For ribs 1-2 the patient turns their head away from the dysfunctional side while flexing into the forearm that is over their forehead.

12. Answer: **B**

This describes the typical technique for muscle energy using post-isometric relaxation which is the typical type of muscle energy that is taught in school. First the restrictive barrier is engaged, the patient contracts against a counterforce with an isometric muscle contraction, the muscle group relaxes, and then a new restrictive barrier is engaged and the technique is repeated.

High Velocity Low Amplitude (HVLA) 16

I. Definition

HVLA is **a passive, direct technique** which uses a rapid (high velocity) therapeutic force of brief duration that travels a short distance (low amplitude) within the anatomic range of motion of a joint, and engages the restrictive barrier in one or more planes of motion to elicit release of the restriction.[32 p.1097] The HVLA technique is performed by positioning a restricted joint against its restrictive barrier and applying a short (low amplitude) quick (high velocity) thrust to move the joint past the restrictive barrier. HVLA techniques may also be called thrust techniques.

II. Neurophysiologic mechanism of HVLA

There are 2 theories:

Theory #1 - An HVLA thrust is thought to forcefully stretch a contracted muscle, producing a barrage of afferent impulses from the muscle spindles to the central nervous system. The central nervous system reflexively sends inhibitory impulses to the muscle spindle to relax the muscle. [7 p.306]

Theory #2 -An HVLA thrust is thought to forcefully stretch the contracted muscle pulling on its tendon activiating the Golgi tendon receptors and reflexively relaxing the muscle. [7 p.292]

III. <u>General Procedure:</u>

1. After correct diagnosis of a somatic dysfunction, the physician will move the dysfunctional segment in such a way that it is against its restrictive barrier. This is ideally done by reversing all three planes of motion.

   For example, if a segment was FR_LS_L, the physician would extend, rotate and sidebend the spine to the right (ER_RS_R) until motion is felt at the level of the dysfunctional segment.

   NOTE: Due to the facet orientation and biomechanics in certain regions of the spine, it is not always possible to reverse all three planes of motion (i.e. the cervical spine). See specific HVLA techniques for details.

2. The patient then is asked to relax.

   If the patient is not relaxed, the treatment will fail and the corrective thrust may cause soft tissue damage. The exhalation phase of respiration is the relaxation phase, and the final force is often applied during exhalation. [1 p.672]

3. The physician then uses a short, quick thrust to move the dysfunctional segment through the restrictive barrier. Often, a pop or click is heard along with an increase in the range of motion.

   Be sure to remain against the restrictive barrier before applying the thrust, do not back off before the thrust.

4. Re-evaluate range of motion.

IV. <u>Indications and Contraindications</u>

A. <u>Indications</u>

1. <u>Treatment of motion loss in somatic dysfunction.</u>

   HVLA in general is used to restore motion in previously mobile joints; it is not ordinarily indicated for treatment of joint restriction due to pathologic changes such as contractures or advanced degenerative joint disease. [32 p.360]

B. <u>Absolute contraindications</u> [1, 32, 7]

1. Osteoporosis
2. Osteomyelitis, fractures or bone metastases in the area of thrust
3. Joint instability (i.e. patients with severe rheumatoid arthritis, or Down syndrome, the transverse ligament of the dens may weaken, resulting in atlantal-axial subluxation). HVLA manipulation may lead to rupture of this ligament resulting in catastrophic neurologic damage. [7 p.295]
4. Severe herniated nucleus propulsus with radiculopathy
5. Joint replacement in the area of thrust
6. Vertebrobasilar insufficiency
7. Joint (including vertebral) ankylosis

C. Relative contraindications [1, 32, 7]

1. Mild to moderate strain in the area of thrust (i.e. acute whiplash)
2. Pregnancy
3. Post-surgical conditions
4. Mild to moderate herniated nucleus propulsus with radiculopathy
5. Patients on anticoagulation therapy or hemophiliacs should be treated with great caution to prevent bleeding.
6. Osteoarthritic joints with moderate motion loss

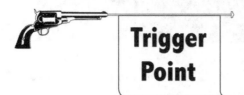

Trigger Point

Know the absolute and relative contraindications for HVLA.

VI. Specific HVLA treatments

A. Cervical
OA FS$_R$R$_L$ (see Fig. 16.1)

1. The patient supine and the physician at the head of the table.
2. Grasp the patient's head and flex the neck slightly.
3. The MCP joint of the thrusting hand is placed at the base of the occiput.
4. Extend the occiput slightly, make sure that extension is limited to only the OA joint.
5. Sidebend the occiput to the left and rotate it to the right to engage the restrictive barrier.
6. Apply a HVLA thrust by translating the occiput to the right. The direction of the thrust should be directed toward the patient's opposite (right) eye.
7. Re-evaluate the range of motion.

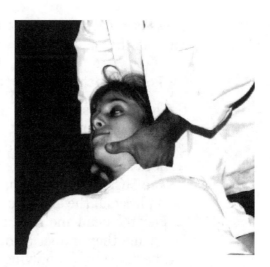

Fig. 16.1: *Treatment of OA FR$_L$S$_R$.*

AA rotated right (AAR$_R$) (see Fig. 16.2)

1. The patient supine and the physician at the head of the table.
2. The palm of the physician's left hand grasps the patient's chin.
3. The index finger of the physician's right hand is placed by the soft tissue of the AA joint. The physician's right thumb contacts the patient's right zygomatic process, avoiding the right mandible.
4. The patient is asked to inhale, then exhale fully.
5. At the end of exhalation, the physician applies a left rotational high velocity, low amplitude thrust using the right index finger as a fulcrum
6. Re-evaluate the range of motion.

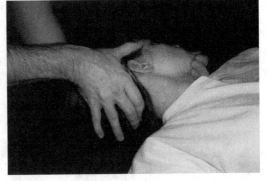

Fig. 16.2: *Treatment of the AA rotated right.*

Typical cervical segments (C2 - C7)

These cervical segments can be treated by using either a sidebending or rotatory thrust.

C3 FS$_L$R$_L$ Rotational thrust (see Fig. 16.3)

1. The patient supine and the physician at the head of the table.
2. Grasp the patient's head and flex the neck slightly.
3. The MCP joint of the thrusting hand is placed at the articular pillar of C3.
4. Flex the head and neck down to C3 and then induce a small amount of extension by applying anterior translation at C3.
5. Rotate the head and neck to the right to the restrictive barrier. Right sidebending is achieved by keeping the patient's right temple close to the table.
6. Apply a right rotatory HVLA thrust using the left MCP as a fulcrum. The direction of the thrust should be directed toward the patient's opposite eye.
7. Re-evaluate the range of motion.

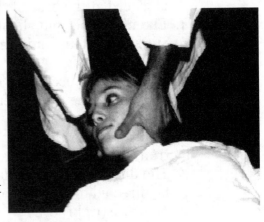

Fig. 16.3: *Treatment of C3 FR$_L$S$_L$, with a rotational thrust.*

C6 ES$_R$R$_R$ Sidebending thrust (see fig 16.4)

1. The patient supine and the physician at the head of the table.
2. The MCP joint of the left hand is placed at the articular pillar of C6.
3. Grasp the patient's head and flex the neck to the C6 - C7 joint. Induce a small amount of extension by applying anterior translation at C6
4. Sidebend the neck to the left until localized at the C6-C7 joint.
5. Rotate the neck to the right to limit motion of (lock) the above facets.
6. Apply a sidebending HVLA thrust by translating C6 to the right. The direction of the thrust should be directed toward the patient's opposite shoulder.
7. Re-evaluate the range of motion.

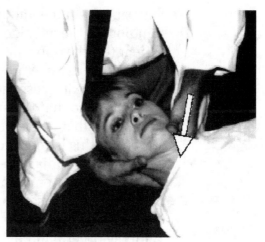

Fig. 16.4: *Treatment of C6 ES$_R$R$_R$, with a sidebending thrust.*

B. Thoracic and ribs

The thoracic segments and ribs can be treated with HVLA in many positions. The position most commonly taught at osteopathic medical schools has been nicknamed the Kirksville Krunch. This technique is easy to understand and versatile. With very little modification of technique the Kirksville Krunch can treat most thoracic and rib dysfunctions. For other types of thoracic HVLA treatments (prone, seated, etc.), please refer to the Foundations of Osteopathic Medicine, [3] An Osteopathic Approach to Diagnosis and Treatment, [2] or Atlas of Osteopathic Techniques. [32]

Acccording to the Foundations of Osteopatic Medicine, Second Edition (technique not described in the third edition), when treating a flexed lesion, the corrective force will be directed at the dysfunctional segment and the thrust is aimed toward the floor. When treating an extended lesion the corrective thrust is directed at the vertebra below the dysfunctional segment and the thrust is aimed 45° cephalad. A neutral lesion is treated the same way as a flexed dysfunction, however sidebend the patient away from you. A purely flexed or extended lesion (no rotation or sidebending) is treated using roughly the same position, except the physician will use a bilateral fulcrum (thenar eminence under one transverse process and a flexed MCP under the other transverse process). Ribs 2-10 can also be treated using the Kirksville Krunch. The difference is that the physician's thenar eminence is under the posterior rib angle of the "key" rib.

T7 FS$_R$R$_R$ (see Fig. 16.5)

1. The patient supine and the physician standing on the left side of the patient (on the opposite side of the posterior transverse process).
2. The patient will cross their arm over their chest, so that the superior arm is opposite that of the physician. For simplicity this is referred to as "opposite over adjacent."
3. Place the thenar eminence under the posterior transverse process of the dysfunctional segment.
4. With the other hand flex the patient's torso to the T7 -T8 joint space.
5. Sidebend the patient to the left, engaging the restrictive barrier.
6. Have the patient take a deep breath in and exhale.
7. At the end of exhalation, apply an HVLA thrust straight down toward your fulcrum (thenar eminence).

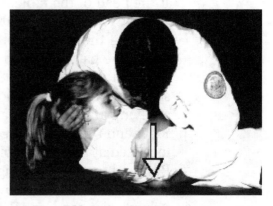

Fig. 16.5: *Treatment of T7 FR$_R$S$_R$. The arrow in the diagram demonstrates the direction of the thrust.*

T7 ES$_R$R$_R$ (see Fig. 16.6)

1. The patient supine and the physician standing on the left side of the patient (on the opposite side of the posterior transverse process).
2. Patient crosses arms across chest, opposite over adjacent.
3. Place the thenar eminence under the posterior transverse process of the vertebra **below** the dysfunctional segment.
4. With the other hand, flex the patient's torso to the T7 -T8 joint space.
5. Sidebend the patient to the left, engaging the restrictive barrier.
6. Have the patient take a deep breath in and exhale.
7. At the end of exhalation, apply an HVLA thrust directed 45° cephalad toward your fulcrum (thenar eminence).

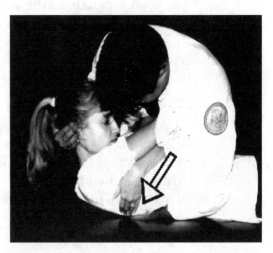

Fig. 16.6: *Treatment for T7 ES$_R$R$_R$. The arrow in the diagram demonstrates the direction of the thrust.*

T7 NS$_L$R$_R$ (see Fig. 16.7)

1. The patient supine and the physician standing on the left side of the patient (on the opposite side of the posterior transverse process).
2. Patient crosses arms opposite over adjacent.
3. Place the thenar eminence under the posterior transverse process of the dysfunctional segment.
4. With the other hand flex the patient's torso to the T7 -T8 joint space.
5. Sidebend the patient to the right (away from you) engaging the restrictive barrier.
6. Have the patient take a deep breath in and exhale.

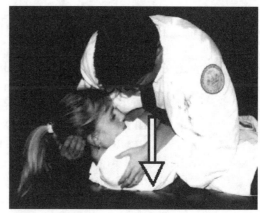

Fig. 16.7: Treatment for T7 NS$_L$R$_R$. Remember to sidebend the patient away from you to engage the barrier.

7. At the end of exhalation, apply an HVLA thrust straight down toward your fulcrum (thenar eminence).

Rib 1 inhalation dysfunction (rib held up)(see fig 16.8)

NOTE: Inhalation dysfunctions of rib one cannot be treated using the Kirksville Krunch.

1. The patient supine and the physician at the head of the table.
2. Sidebend the head and neck to the side of the dysfunctional rib.
3. Rotate the head and neck away.
4. Place the 1st MCP on the tubercle of rib 1.
5. Have the patient take a deep breath in and exhale.
6. At the end ofexhalation, apply an HVLA thrust through the thenar eminence. The direction of the

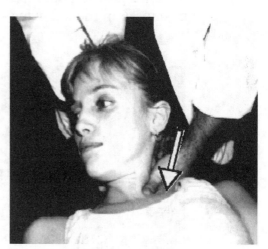

Fig. 16.8: *Treatment for an inhalation dysfunction of rib 1.*

thrust should be posterioanterior and caudad.

Right rib inhalation (rib held up) or exhalation dysfunction (rib held down) (inhalation or exhalation rib or exhalation or inhalation restriction). Kirksville Krunch treatment type (Range: ribs 2- 10).

1. The patient supine and the physician standing on the left side of the patient (stand on the opposite side of the dysfunctional rib).
2. Patient crosses arms opposite over adjacent.
3. Place the thenar eminence under the posterior rib angle of the "key" rib (see Chapter 3 for further explanation of "key" rib).
4. With the other hand flex, the patient's torso and slightly sidebend away from the dysfunctional rib.
5. Have the patient take a deep breath in and exhale.
6. At end exhalation, apply a HVLA thrust straight down toward your fulcrum (thenar eminence).

C. Lumbar Spine

T10-L5 may be treated with HVLA using the "lumbar roll." Flexion, extension or neutral lesions can all be treated in the same lateral recumbent position. The physician may treat the patient with the posterior transverse process up or the posterior transverse process down. For example, if L3 was FRS_R, the physician can treat the patient in the left lateral recumbent position (posterior transverse process up) or in the right lateral recumbent position (transverse process down). There is only one modification with the patient's position between the two treatments. This modification is italicized in step #6 in the following examples and summarized in Table 16.1.

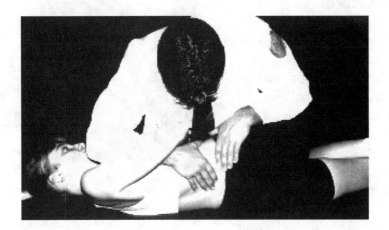

Fig. 16.9: Treatment position for a lumbar roll.

Table 16.1

Lumbar Roll Treatment

Type II Dysfunction:
If treating the patient with the transverse process up => pull the patient's inferior arm down.
If treating the patient with the transverse process down => pull the patient's inferior arm up.

Type I Dysfunction:
If treating the patient with the transverse process up => pull the patient's inferior arm up.
If treating the patient with the transverse process down => pull the patient's inferior arm down.

Type II (flexed or extended) posterior transverse process up
L3 ER$_R$S$_R$

1. Patient in the left lateral recumbent position (posterior transverse process up).
2. Stand in front of the patient.
3. Flex the patient's legs until you palpate motion at L3.
4. Straighten the patient's inferior leg.
5. Hook the superior foot in the lower legs popliteal fossa
6. *Pull patient's inferior arm out (toward you) to rotate the torso and caudad to induce left sidebending down to the dysfunctional segment.*
7. Place one arm in the patient's axilla and the other on the patient's iliac crest.
8. Have the patient take a deep breath in and exhale.
9. At the end of exhalation, apply an HVLA thrust by rotating the patient's pelvis forward and toward the table.
10. Retest the range of motion.

Type II (flexed or extended) posterior transverse process down
L3 ER$_R$S$_R$

1. Patient in the right lateral recumbent position (posterior transverse process down).
2. Stand in front of the patient.
3. Flex the patient's legs until you palpate motion at L3.
4. Straighten the patient's inferior leg.
5. Hook the superior foot in the lower leg's popliteal fossa.
6. *Pull patient's inferior arm out (toward you) to rotate the torso and cephalad to induce left sidebending down to the dysfunctional segment.*
7. Place one arm in the patient's axilla and the other on the patient's iliac crest.
8. Have the patient take a deep breath in and exhale.
9. At the end ofexhalation, apply an HVLA thrust by rotating the patient's pelvis forward and toward the table.
10. Retest the range of motion.

NOTE: Flexion or extension can also be added to further engage another barrier. With the patient in the lateral recumbent position, anterior motion of the torso will produce flexion, posterior motion will produce extension.

Type I (neutral dysfunctions) posterior transverse process up
L3 NS$_L$R$_R$

1. Patient in the left lateral recumbent position (posterior transverse process up).
2. Stand in front of the patient.
3. Flex the patient's legs until you palpate motion at L3.
4. Straighten the patient's inferior leg.
5. Hook the superior foot in the lower leg's popliteal fossa.
6. *Pull patient's inferior arm out (toward you) to rotate the torso and cephalad to induce right sidebending down to the dysfunctional segment.*
7. Place one arm in the patient's axilla and the other on the patient's iliac crest.
8. Have the patient take a deep breath in and exhale.
9. At the end of exhalation, apply an HVLA thrust by rotating the patient's pelvis forward and toward the table.
10. Retest the range of motion.

Type I (neutral dysfunctions) posterior transverse process down
L3 NS$_L$R$_R$

1. Patient in the right lateral recumbent position (posterior transverse process down).
2. Stand in front of the patient.
3. Flex the patient's legs until you palpate motion at L3
4. Straighten the patient's inferior leg.
5. Hook the superior foot in the lower leg's popliteal fossa.
6. *Pull patient's inferior arm out (toward you) to rotate the torso and down caudad to induce right sidebending down to the dysfunctional segment.*
7. Place one arm in the patient's axilla and the other on the patient's iliac crest.
8. Have the patient take a deep breath in and exhale.
9. At the end of exhalation, apply an HVLA thrust by rotating the patient's pelvis forward and toward the table.
10. Retest the range of motion.

Chapter 16 Review Questions

1. A 75-year-old male presents with neck pain. History reveals he recently received HVLA treatment to the cervical spine. Physical examination reveals dizziness when his head is passively rotated and extended. Radiographs reveal moderate degenerative changes of the cervical spine. Compression of which of the following structures is the most likely cause of this patient's symptoms?

   A. brachiocephalic vein
   B. cervical ganglia of sympathetic trunk
   C. nucleus pulposus of the C3-C4 disk
   D. vertebral artery
   E. zygapophysial joint

2. A 25-year-old male presents with neck pain and requests osteopathic manipulation. A history of which of the following would be most contraindicated to performing HVLA in this patient?

   A. joint instability
   B. fibromyalgia
   C. herniated nucleus pulposus without radiculopathy
   D. osteoarthritis
   E. quadriparesis

3. A 25-year-old male complains of back pain and structural examination reveals that T6 is restricted in right rotation. Flexing the body down to T6 causes the segment to further rotate to the left naturally, while extending the area causes T6 to return to the neutral position. The patient is placed in position for the Kirksville Krunch technique. Hand placement should be such that your thenar eminence contacts the

   A. left transverse process of T6
   B. left transverse process of T7
   C. posterior aspect of rib 6
   D. right transverse process of T6
   E. right transverse process of T7

<u>Questions 4-5 refer to the following</u>:

A 34-year-old male presents with neck pain after a motor vehicle accident. You notice that C3 is restricted in left rotation and left sidebending. Rotation improves with flexion and becomes restricted in extension.

4. When using HVLA to treat this somatic dysfunction, you should

    A. only use rotation when performing this technique
    B. rotate the patient's head to the left and sidebend left
    C. rotate the patient's head to the left and sidebend right
    D. rotate the patient's head to the right and sidebend left
    E. rotate the patient's head to the right and sidebend right

5. When performing this technique using a rotational thrust corrective force, it is important to

    A. direct the corrective thrust toward the patient's opposite shoulder
    B. direct the corrective thrust toward the patient's opposite eye
    C. place the segment into extreme flexion
    D. position the segment in the position of ease
    E. rotate and sidebend the segment in opposite directions

<u>Questions 6-7 refer to the following</u>:

A 50-year-old male complains of low back pain. History reveals it is worse when extending backwards. Structural examination reveals the right transverse process of L2 becomes more posterior with extension. The patient is placed in postition for an HVLA treatment so that the patient lying on his left side.

6. During this technique the physician will

    A. position L2 in a sidebent left position
    B. introduce extension by flexing the patients legs up to L2
    C. introduce extension by flexing the patient's torso down to L2
    D. move the patient's bent legs cephalad until motion is felt at the L1 interspinous space
    E. flex L2 in relation to L3

7. The final corrective thrust emphasizes

    A. rotation
    B. distraction of L2 left
    C. inhalation
    D. flexion
    E. sidebending

<u>Questions 8-9 refer to the following</u>:

A 30-year-old presents with sacroiliac pain. Structural examination reveals a positive seated flexion test on the right, anterior motion restriction at the left lower pole, a deep right sacral sulcus with associated tissue texture changes and tenderness to palpation and L5 rotated right.

8. Which of the following best describes the sacral dysfunction

    A. Right on right sacral torsion
    B. Unilateral sacral flexion on the left
    C. Posterior sacrum left
    D. Left on left sacral torsion
    E. Unilateral sacral flexion on the right

9. The patient consents to osteopathic manipulation using HVLA. The corrective force should be directed at:

    A. The left inferior lateral angle
    B. L5
    C. The left sacral sulcus
    D. The left sacroiliac joint
    E. The right sacral sulcus

Explanations

1. Answer: **D**

    There are several risks involved with performing HVLA and one must understand the regional anatomy to appreciate these risks. Severe neurovascular accidents can be associated with upper cervical manipulation, such as vertebral artery compression with thrombosis, occipitobasilar strokes (Wallenberg syndrome), arterial dissections, or cerebellar infarctions. These primarily occur with use of rotational forces with the head extended, thereby compressing or manipulating the vertebral artery within the transverse foramen.

2. Answer: **A**

    Joint instability such as those patients with rheumatoid arthritis and Down syndrome are at risk during direct cervical manipulation because of the odontoid ligament weakening and susceptibility to rupture causing a spinal cord injury. Complications such as fracture are associated with the following underlying conditions: osteoporosis, metastatic bone disease, bone infections, vertebral tuberculosis. A severe disc herniation with radiculopathy is an absolute contraindication, however a mild to moderate disc herniation without radiculopathy is a relative contraindication.

3. Answer: **E**

    This patient has a T6 that is ER_LS_L. Somatic dysfunction is named for the freedom of motion, thus the T6 segment is rotated left and is restricted in right rotation. The segment is also more free with extension as it is described as returning more to neutral position with this motion. Thus T6, is now known to be flexed and rotated left. Since T6 demonstrates non-neutral mechanics (flexed or extended), it follows Fryette type II mechanics where the segment sidebends and rotates in the same direction. When treating this with HVLA using the Kirksville Krunch technique, the thenar eminence is placed under the posterior transverse process of the vertebrae below the dysfunctional segment (in this case T7).

4. Answer: **B**

    Recall that somatic dysfunction is named for the freedom of motion. The patient has C3 that is flexed, rotated and sidebent right. HVLA is a direct technique and because of this the affected segment should be put into the restrictive barrier . C3 should be rotated left and sidebent left.

5. Answer: **B**

    When using a rotary corrective thrust, it should be directed toward the patients opposite eye. A sidebending thrust is directed toward the patient's opposite shoulder.

6. Answer: **A**

    The patient has L2 flexed, rotated and sidebent right. In this patient, the right transverse process of L2 becomes more posterior with extension. Therefore, L2 is likely flexed and rotated right. Since the asymmetry worsens with extension, Fryette's type II mechanics apply, and L2 must sidebend in the same direction of rotation. In order to apply HVLA (which is a direct technique), L2 must be positioned in a sidebent left position. Flexing the patient's legs up to L2 or flexion of the patient's torso down to L2 will induce flexion, not extension. The patient's bent legs should be moved cephalad until motion is felt at the L2/3 interspinous space. Since the segment is flexed, the segment should be treated in an extended position using a direct technique.

7. Answer: **E**

    The final corrective thrust involves rotating the patient's pelvis forward toward the practitioner while maitaining the patients upper torso in the supine position. This is done at end exhalation, not during patient inhalation. The final thrust for a lumbar HVLA technique does ot involve distraction, flexion or sidebending.

8. Answer: **D**

    This patient has a left on left sacral torsion (left rotation on a left oblique axis). It is similar to an anterior right sacrum. Structural exam will reveal a deep right sacral sulcus, positive seated flexion test on the right,, and restriction of springing (anterior motion) on the left ILA (left lower pole). In a sacral torsion, L5 rotates in the opposite direction of the sacrum.

9. Answer: **B**

    As a general rule, L5 is treated prior to treating sacral dyfunctions. See Chapter 6 "Sacrum and Innominates"

Articulatory Techniques

17

I. <u>Definition</u>

Articulatory techniques (also called springing techniques or low velocity/moderate amplitude techniques) are direct techniques that increase range of motion in a restricted joint. The physician engages the restrictive barrier and uses gentle repetitive forces to increase range of motion within that joint.[61 p. 765] Respiratory cooperation and/or muscle energy activation are frequently added to further stretch tight myofascial structures that may limit articular motion.

Post-operative patients and elderly patients find articulatory techniques more acceptable than other vigorous types of direct techniques, since articulating forces are gentle in nature. [1 p.765]

A. <u>Indications:</u>

1. Limited or lost articular motion
2. Need to increase frequency or amplitude of motion of a body region. For example, the need to increase frequency and amplitude of chest wall motion in a person with respiratory disease.
3. The need to normalize sympathetic activity (rib raising technique)

B. <u>Contraindications:</u>[1 p.765]

1. Repeated rotation of the upper cervical spine when positioned in extension may cause damage to the vertebral artery.
2. Acutely inflamed joint especially where the cause of the inflammation may be from an infection or fracture.

C. Typical articulatory procedure

1. Move the affected joint to the limit of all ranges of motion. Once a restrictive barrier is reached slowly and firmly, continue to apply gentle force against it.
2. At this time you may use respiratory cooperation or muscle energy activation to further increase myofascial stretch of tight tissues.
3. Return the articulation to its neutral position.
4. Repeat the process several times.
5. Cease repetition of motion when no further response is achieved.

II. Frequently used articulatory techniques

A. Rib raising

Purpose:

1. Increase chest wall motion.
2. Normalize sympathetic activity.[7 p.57, 20 p.69]
   The thoracic chain ganglia lie directly anterior to the corresponding rib heads. Movement of the chain ganglia by rib raising initially stimulates the sympathetic outflow, but this is followed by long-lasting sympathetic inhibition.
3. Improve lymphatic return.
   Rib raising is useful for those patients who have a resistant or noncompliant chest wall, such as a patient with viral pneumonia. Since pneumonia (as well as other disease processes [7 p.73]) is associated with hypersympathetic activity, **rib raising will normalize this sympathetic hyperactivity**. Rib raising can be done in the seated or supine position. The supine position is described here.

Procedure: [32 p.525]

1. Patient supine.
2. Physician seated at the side of the patient.
3. Place your hands under the patient's thorax, contacting the rib angles with the pads of your fingers.
4. Apply gentle traction.
5. Raise the patients ribs by pushing your fingertips anteriorly and lowering your forearms (It is easier to push your fingers anteriorly by using your forearm as a lever).

B. <u>Spencer techniques</u> (Seven Stages of Spencer)

This technique is useful in patients who have developed fibrosis and restriction during a period of inactivity (adhesive capsulitis) following an injury. Such injuries may include a healed rotator cuff tear, or immobilization of the shoulder girdle after a humerus fracture.

The Spencer techniques are performed in 7 stages. In all stages, the patient is in the lateral recumbent position lying with the side of the dysfunctional shoulder up. The physician stands on the side of the table facing the patient, then carefully and slowly moves the upper extremity through the following sequence: [1 p. 779-782]

<u>Stage I:</u> Glenohumeral extension with elbow flexed

<u>Stage II:</u> Glenohumeral flexion with the elbow extended

<u>Stage III:</u> Circumduction with slight compression and elbow flexed

<u>Stage IV:</u> Circumduction with slight traction and elbow extended

<u>Stage V:</u> Broken in to two parts:

   Va: Adduction and external rotation with the elbow flexed

   Vb: Abduction and internal rotation with the elbow flexed

<u>Stage VI:</u> Abduction and internal rotation with arm behind the back

<u>Stage VII:</u> Traction with inferior glide

<u>NOTE</u>: The purpose of this technique is to improve motion in the glenohumoral joint, therefore, it is important that the physician limits motion at the scapula by placing his hand on the top of the patient's shoulder. Muscle energy techniques can also be utilized at each of the shoulder's restrictive barriers.

Chapter 17 Review Questions

1. A elderly male status post lumbar laminectomy 6 weeks ago complains of low back pain and is observed ambulating in a forward flexed position. Standing examination reveals a positive side shift to the right. X-rays demonstrate no fracture, but notable facet arthropathy at the level of the L4/5 surgical side. The patient elects to undergo a low velocity/moderate amplitude technique. What clinical considerations are important when choosing this technique in this scenerio? Low velocity/moderate amplitude techniques:

    A. are not indicated to restore motion to facet joints
    B. tend to be strenuous and are typically not suitable for elderly patients
    C. tend to be generally well tolerated on post operative patients.
    D. always require active patient participation
    E. is indirect and therefore the restrictive barrier is not engaged

2. An elderly female just had open reduction, internal fixation of her hip after a fracture and is now stabilizing on post-operative day 2. Multiple somatic dysfunctions of the thoracic region and ribs are discovered and the provider elects to use rib raising to encourage recovery. Which is most associated with this technique?

    A. an increase of sympathetic activity typically occurrs after an initial decrease
    B. it is a useful technique in patients with viral pneumonia
    C. it must be performed during inhalation because the ribs fall during exhalation
    D. it must be performed in the prone position
    E. the technique is autonomic in nature and has little or no effect on chest wall motion

Questions 3-6 refer to the following:

A 55-year-old female presents with chronic shoulder pain in her non-dominant arm. History reveals she injured the shoulder several years ago at work and never sought out care for this. Subsequently she has used the arm less and less throughout the years secondary to worsening pain. After informed consent the patient elects for non-operative treatment with physical therapy and the Spencer technique.

3. Stage 1 involves glenohumeral

    A. abduction with the elbow extended
    B. adduction with the elbow extended
    C. extension with the elbow flexed
    D. flexion with the elbow flexed
    E. internal rotation with the elbow flexed

4. Stage 2 involves glenohumeral

   A. abduction with the elbow extended
   B. adduction with the elbow extended
   C. extension with the elbow flexed
   D. flexion with the elbow extended
   E. circumduction and traction

5. Stage 3 primarily tests the

   A. articular surface
   B. joint capsule
   C. radial head
   D. radioulnar joint
   E. rotator cuff tendons

6. Stage 4 primarily tests the

   A. articular surface
   B. joint capsule
   C. radial head
   D. radioulnar joint
   E. rotator cuff tendons

7. Stage 5 involves glenohumeral

   A. abduction with internal rotation and elbow flexed
   B. adduction with internal and external rotation and the elbow flexed
   C. extension with the elbow flexed
   D. flexion with the elbow flexed
   E. circumduction and traction

8. Stage 6 places the forearm behind the patient's back with the hand and wrist over
    the "hip pocket" area. This is engaging glenohumeral

   A. adduction
   B. extension
   C. external rotation
   D. flexion
   E. internal rotation

Explanations

1. Answer: **C**

    The patient most likely has iliopsoas hypertonicity on the left or features of psoas syndrome. Low velocity/moderate amplitude techniques are another name for articulatory techniques. These techniques are usually more gentle direct techniques that engage the restrictive barrier with passive forces. Patient participation in the form of resiratory assistance and muscle energy can sometimes be used during an articulatory treatment. The goal of articultory techniques is to improve range of motion of joints, including facet joints. Post-operative patients and elderly patients find articulatory techniques more acceptable than other vigorous types of direct techniques, since articulating forces are gentle in nature. [1 p.765]

2. Answer: **B**

    Rib raising helps to increase chest wall motion and normalize sympathetic activity. With initial rib raising there will be an initial increase in sympathetic activity folliwed by a sustained decrease in sympathetic activity. With the patient in the supine position the pads of the fingers raise the ribs with gentle traction while contacting the rib angles during patient inhalation and exhalation. The technique is indicated for viral pneumonia. There is good evidence that this and other lymphatic treatments reduce hospitalization and IV antibiotic duration much similar to chest physiotherapy and incentive spirometry. [20 p.280]

3. Answer: **C**

    There are 7 stages to the Spencer technique. During testing and treatment the scapula is fixed in position to permit movement only at the glenohumeral joint. Stage 1 glenohumeral extension with the elbow flexed.

4. Answer: **D**

    Stage 2 involves flexion of the glenohumeral joint with elbow extension.

5. Answer: **A**

    Stage 3 involves circumduction of the upper extremity while applying compression. This motion primarily tests the surface of the glenohumeral joint (labrum and articular surface of the humerus).

6. Answer: **B**

Stage 4 involves circumduction of the upper extremity while applying traction. This motion primarily tests the capsule of the glenohumeral joint.

7. Answer: **A**

Stage V: Is broken into two parts:

Va: Adduction and external rotation with the elbow flexed

Vb: Abduction and internal rotation with the elbow flexed

8. Answer: **E**

Stage 6 involves some abduction but mostly internal rotation of the glenohumeral joint as the elbow is pulled anteriorly.

Special Tests. 18

I. Cervical spine

A. Spurling Test (Compression Test)

Narrowing of the neural foramina can cause referred pain into the ipsilateral arm upon compression of the cervical spine, due to nerve root compression. With the patient seated, the physician extends and sidebends the C-spine to the side being tested, and pushes downward on the top of the patient's head. The test is positive if pain radiates into the ipsilateral arm. The pain's distribution can help localize the affected nerve root.[23 p.50-51, 24 p.127, 24 p.411]

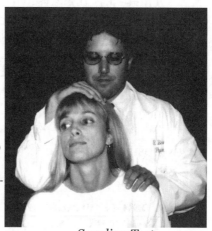

Spurling Test

B. Wallenberg Test

To test for vertebral artery insufficiency, in a supine position the physician flexes the patient's neck, holding it for ten seconds, then extends the neck holding it for ten seconds. The same is done for head and neck rotation to the right and left, head and neck rotation right and left with the neck in the extended position, and in positions that the physician would attempt to mobilize the C-spine. A positive test results when the patient complains of dizziness, visual changes, lightheadedness, or eye nystagmus occurs. [23 p.53-54]

It is important to detect vertebral artery insufficiency, as a result similar tests to Wallenberg test have been described in the medical literature. These tests are essentially variations of Wallenberg test. One particular test that has been described in the osteopathic literature is **Underberg test**. This test is perfomed with the neck backward bent and the head fully rotated to either side. If the patient develops vascular or neurologic symptoms, HVLA is contraindicated. [7 p.586]

II. Shoulder

A. Thoracic Outlet Syndrome Tests

1. Adson Test

The neurovascular bundle can be compromised by tight scalene muscles. While monitoring the patient's pulse, the arm is extended at the elbow, the shoulder is extended, externally rotated, and slightly abducted. The patient is then asked to take a deep breath and turn his/her head toward the ipsilateral arm. The test is positive with a severely decreased or absent radial pulse. [24 p.127, 23 p.122, 7 p.528]

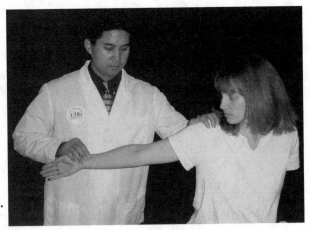

Adson's test

2. Wright's test [23 p.120] (a.k.a. arm hyperextension test)[7 p.529]

This neurovascular bundle can be compromised as it passes under the pectoralis minor muscle at the coracoid process. This test entails hyperabducting the arm above the head with some extension. The test is positive with a severely decreased or absent radial pulse.

3. Costoclavicular syndrome test [23 p.122] (a.k.a. Military Posture Test)[7 p.528]

The neurovascular bundle can be compromised between the clavicle and the first rib. The examiner palpates the radial pulse while depressing and extending the shoulder. The test is positive with a severely decreased or absent radial pulse.

B. Apley scratch test

This test is used to evaluate the range of motion of the shoulder. To test abduction and external rotation, ask the patient to reach behind the head and touch the opposite shoulder. To evaluate internal rotation and adduction, ask the patient to reach in front of the head and touch the opposite shoulder. Next, to further evaluate internal rotation and adduction, instruct the patient to reach behind the back and touch the inferior angle of the opposite scapula. Observe the patient's movement for any asymmetry or any limitations of movement.

Another way to evaluate range of motion of both shoulders at once is to ask the patient to abduct the arms to 90°, then supinate the forearms and continue abduction until the hands touch overhead. This will compare bilateral abduction. Next, to test abduction and external rotation, ask the patient to interlock the hands behind the head and push the elbows posteriorly. Finally, instruct the patient to place the hands behind the back as high as possible as if to touch the ipsilateral inferior angle of the scapula.[1 p.649, 24 p.21]

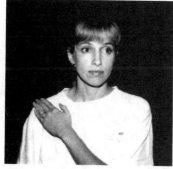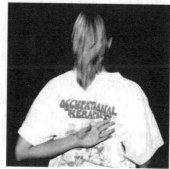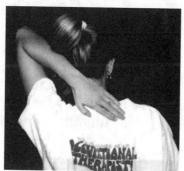

C. Drop Arm Test

This test detects tears in the rotator cuff. The patient is instructed to abduct the shoulder to 90°, and then to slowly lower the arm. A positive test results if the patient cannot lower the arm smoothly, or if the arm drops to the side from 90°. [1 p.649, 23 p.118]

D. Speed Test

This test assesses the biceps tendon in the bicipital groove. The patient fully extends the elbow, flexes the shoulder and supinates the forearm. The physician resists the flexion of the shoulder. A positive test occurs with tenderness in the bicipital groove. [23 p.117]

E. Yergason Test

This test determines the stability of the biceps tendon in the bicipital groove. The patient flexes the elbow to 90° while the physician grasps the elbow with one hand and the wrist with the other hand. While pulling downward on the patient's elbow, the physician externally rotates the forearm as the patient resists this motion. A positive test results when pain is elicited as the biceps tendon pops out of the bicipital groove. [24 p. 32, 23 p.117]

III. Wrist

A. Allen Test

This test assesses the adequacy of blood supply to the hand by the radial and ulnar arteries. The patient is instructed to open and close the hand being tested several times and then to make a tight fist. The physician occludes the radial and ulnar arteries at the wrist. The patient is then asked to open the hand; the palm should be pale. The physician releases one of the arteries and assesses the flushing of the hand. If it flushes slowly, or not at all, then the released artery is not adequately supplying the hand. This procedure is repeated for the other artery. [24 p.102-3]

B. Finkelstein Test

To test for tenosynovitis in the abductor pollicis longus and extensor pollicis brevis tendons at the wrist (De Quervain disease), the patient makes a fist with the thumb tucked inside the fingers. The physician stabilizes the patient's forearm and deviates the wrist ulnarly. A positive test results when the patient feels pain over the tendons at the wrist.[23 p.189; 24 p.76-77]

C. Phalen Test

This test aides in the diagnosis of carpal tunnel syndrome. The physician maximally flexes the patient's wrist and holds this position for one minute. If a "tingling" sensation is felt in the thumb, index finger, middle and lateral portion of the ring fingers, the test is positive and is indicative of carpal tunnel syndrome. [24 p.83, 23 p.194]

D. Reverse Phalen's Test (Prayer test)

Also used in the diagnosis of carpal tunnel syndrome, this test has the patient extend the wrist while gripping the physician's hand. If after one minute, the same symptoms are seen as in Phalen test, the reverse Phalen test is positive. [23 p.194]

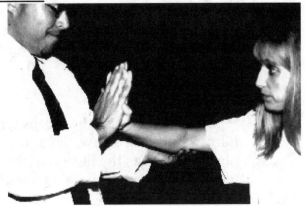

Reverse Phalen Test

E. Tinel Test

This test is used in the diagnosis of carpal tunnel syndrome. The physician taps over the volar aspect of the patient's transverse carpal ligament. A positive test will cause tingling or paresthesia into the thumb, index, middle and lateral half of the ring finger. [23. p.194, 24 p.82]

NOTE: Tinel test may also be used in the diagnosis of other neuropathies, such as ulnar nerve entrapment at the elbow, peroneal compression at the fibular head and posterior tibial nerve entrapment at the ankle. [24 p.57, 23 p.484]

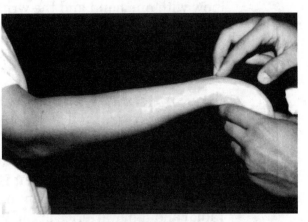

Tinel test at the wrist

IV. Lumbar spine

A. Hip-drop Test

This test assesses the sidebending ability of the lumbar spine and thoracolumbar junction. With the patient standing, the physician locates the most superior and lateral aspect of the iliac crests. The patient is instructed to bend one knee without lifting the heel from the floor. Normally, the lumber spine should sidebend toward the side contralateral to the bending knee, producing a smooth convexity in the lumbar spine on the ipsilateral side. The ipsilateral iliac crest should drop more than 20-25°. A positive test is indicated by anything less than a smooth convexity in the lumbar spine, or a drop of the iliac crest of less than 20-25°, and alerts the physician to a somatic dysfunction of the lumbar or the thoracolumbar spine.[1 p.426]

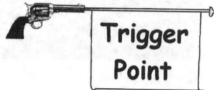

Trigger Point

The purpose of the hip-drop test is to evaluate sidebending (lateral flexion) of the lumbar spine

B. Straight Leg Raising Test (Lasegue Test)

This test is used in the evaluation of sciatic nerve compression. The patient lies supine. The physician grasps the leg being tested under the heel with the hand, and to keep the knee extended, places the other hand on the anterior aspect of the knee. The physician then lifts the leg upward, flexing the hip. The leg is lifted until the patient feels discomfort. Normally, the leg can be raised to about 70-80° of hip flexion.

If the patient experiences pain, the most likely cause will be due to hamstring tightness or due to problems with the sciatic nerve. Once the patient feels pain upon lifting the leg, the physician lowers the leg just beyond where the pain was felt, and then dorsiflexes the foot (Braggard Test). This stretches the sciatic nerve. If no pain is elicited, the pain from the leg-raising is probably from tight hamstrings and the test is considered negative. If pain is felt all the way down the leg, this indicates a sciatic origin, and the straight leg raising test is considered positive. [23 p.267, 24 p.256]

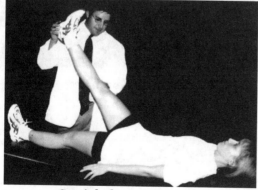

Straight leg raising test

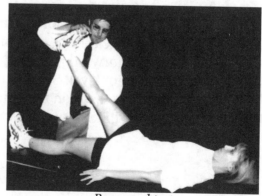

Braggard test

V. Sacrum and Innominates

A. Seated Flexion Test

This test assesses sacroiliac motion. It evaluates somatic dysfunction in the pelvis, most commonly in the sacrum. [1 p.428] The patient is seated with both feet flat on the floor. The physician locates the patient's PSIS's and places his thumbs on the inferior notch. The patient is instructed to bend forward and the physician assesses the level of the PSIS's as this motion is completed. A positive test occurs when, at the termination of forward bending, the PSIS's are not level. Somatic dysfunction is present on the side of the superior PSIS.

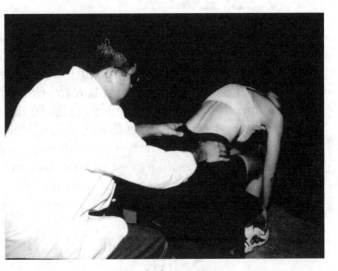

Seated Flexion Test

B. Standing Flexion Test

This test assesses **iliosacral motion**. It evaluates the possibility of somatic dysfunction in the leg or pelvis, most commonly the innominate. [1 p.428] With the patient standing, the physician locates the patient's PSIS's and places his thumbs on the inferior notch. The patient is instructed to bend forward and the physician assesses the level of the PSIS's as this motion is completed. A positive test occurs when, at the termination of forward bending, the PSIS's are not level. Somatic dysfunction is present on the side of the superior PSIS.

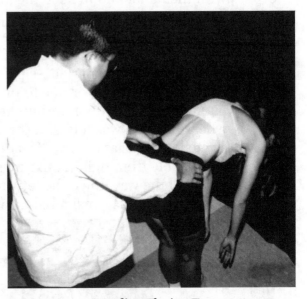

Standing Flexion Test

C. ASIS Compression Test

This test helps determine the side of a SI dysfunction. It is particularly helpful when the standing or seated flexion tests are equivocal. With the patient in the supine position, the physician comes in contact with the ASIS's and applies a posterior compression to each ASIS while stabilizing the other. There is usually an ease of posterior compression (some authors [7] describe this as a sense of "resiliency"). If there is a resistance to compression (that side did not have "resiliency") then the test is considered positive on that side. A positive test indicates dysfunction of the sacrum, innominate or pubic bones. [1 p.588]

D. Pelvic side shift test [1 p.592]

This test determines if the sacrum is in the midline. With the patient standing, the physician stabilizes the shoulders with the right hand and pushes the pelvis to the right with the left hand. The hands are then switched and the pelvis is translated to the left. The test is positive on the side of freer translation. This indicates that the pelvis is shifted to that side.

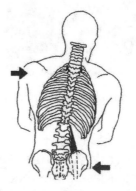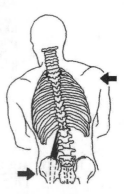

Positive pelvic shift test to the left.   *Positive pelvic shift test to the right.*

It is often seen in a flexion contracture of the iliopsoas (psoas syndrome). A flexion contacture of the right iliopsoas will cause a positive pelvic shift test to the left and vice versa. It can also be caused from postural imbalance such as a short leg. [1 p.592, 7 p. 486]

E. Trendelenberg's Test

This test assesses gluteus medius muscle strength. The physician stands behind the patient. The patient is instructed to pick one of the legs up off the floor. Normally, the gluteus medius muscle should pull up the unsupported pelvis to keep it level. A positive test occurs when the pelvis falls, which indicates weakness in the gluteus medius muscle. [23 p.323, 24 p.164] For example if the patient is standing on the left leg and their right pelvis falls, this indicated weakness in the left gluteus medius muscle.

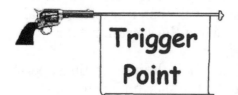

Trigger Point

The Trendelenberg Test indicated weakness of the gluteus medius muscle on the leg that the patient is standing on.

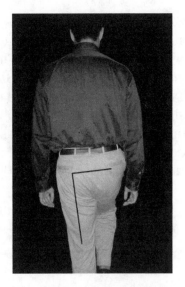 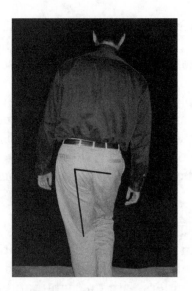

Negative Trendelenberg   *Positive Trendelenberg indicates left gluteus medius weakness*

F   Spring test (a.k.a. lumbosacral spring test) [1 p.1109]

This test assesses whether or not the sacral base is tilted posterior. With the patient in the prone position, the physician will place the heel of the hand over the lumbosacral junction. Gentle and rapid springing is applied downward onto the lumbosacral junction. The test is positive when there is little or no springing. This is indicative of the sacral base moving posteriorly. This test is postive in a unilateral sacral extension, sacral margin posterior, sacral base posterior and when the sacrum rotates backward on an oblique axis

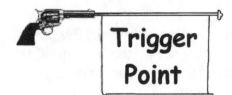

Trigger Point

The spring test will be positive in all the dysfunctions in which the sacral base moves posterior.

G. Backward bending test [1 p. 598, 1089] **(a.k.a. The Sphinx Test)**

This test determines if the sacral base has moved posterior or anterior. The test is positive if a part of the sacral base moves posterior (a unilateral sacral extension, sacral margin posterior and when the sacrum rotates backward on an oblique axis).

With the patient prone, the physician places their thumbs on the superior sulci. If asymmetry is present, either one side of the sacrum has moved posterior, or the other side has moved anterior. To determine between the two, have the patient prop up on their elbows (sphinx position). Normally, this movement (lumbar extension) causes the sacral base to move anteriorly. If one side of the sacral base is anterior, it will move more anteriorly with lumbar extension and consequently the physician's thumbs will become more symmetrical. However, if part of the sacral base is posterior, it will resist anterior movement with lumbar extension and consequently the physician's thumbs will become more asymmetric.

- *If the physician's thumbs become more symmetric with lumbar extension, part of the sacral base moved anterior.*
- *If the physician's thumbs become more asymmetric with lumbar extension, part of the sacral base has moved posterior.*

VI. <u>Hips</u>

A. <u>Ober Test</u>

This test detects a tight tensor fascia lata and iliotibial band. The patient lies on the side opposite the iliotibial band being tested. The physician stands behind the patient and flexes the knee on the side being tested to 90°, abducts the hip as far as possible, and slightly extends the hip while stabilizing the pelvis to keep the patient from rolling. Slight hip extension is necessary to ensure that the iliotibial band passes directly over the greater trochanter. The physician slowly allows the thigh to fall to the table. The test is positive if the thigh remains in the abducted position, indicating a tight iliotibial band. [23 p.354, 24 p.167]

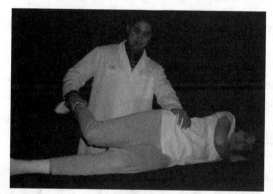

Negative Ober test

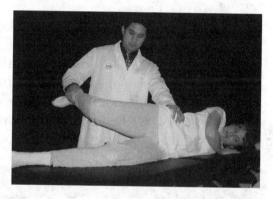

Positive Ober test

B. Patrick Test (FABERE Test)

This test is used to assess pathology of the sacroiliac and hip joint, especially osteoarthritis of the hip. The term FABERE indicates the positioning of the hip being tested. Flexion, Abduction, External Rotation, then Extension. The patient's hip is flexed, abducted, and externally rotated into a figure-4 position. Any pain in or around the hip joint indicates general pathology of that hip joint. At this point, the physician places one hand on the contralateral ASIS and the other hand on the knee of the testing leg. Pressure is placed downward on both points, the most important motion being the further extension of the hip. Pain will be accentuated by any arthritic changes in the hip or sacroiliac joint. [1 p.607, 23 p. 343, 24 p.262]

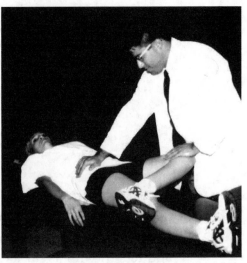

Patrick Test

C. Thomas Test

This test assesses the possibility of a flexion contracture of the hip, usually of iliopsoas origin. The patient lies supine and the physician checks for exaggerated lumbar lordosis, common in hip flexion contractures. The physician flexes one hip so that knee and anterior thigh touches the patient's abdomen. If a flexion contracture is not present, the patient's opposite leg will remain flat on the table. If present, a contracture of the iliopsoas will cause the opposite leg to lift off of the table. [23 p.152, 24 p.155]

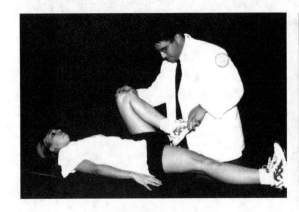

Negative Thomas Test

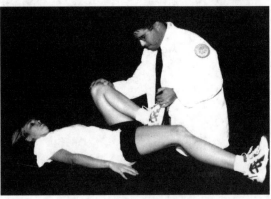

Positive Thomas Test

VII. Knee

A. Anterior and Posterior Drawer Tests

These tests are used to assess the anterior and posterior cruciate ligaments. The patient lies supine with the hip flexed to 45° and knee flexed to 90°. The physician sits on the patient's foot of the knee being tested, wraps both hands around behind the tibia, and places one thumb on the medial joint line and one on the lateral joint line. The tibia is then pulled anteriorly (anterior drawer) to test the ACL. If the tibia slides out from under the femur, the test is positive for an ACL tear. Both sides must be compared because some movement may be possible in some patients. The physician then pushes posteriorly on the tibia to check the PCL (posterior drawer). After comparing both knees, the test is positive if the tibia excessively moves backward under the femur. [1 p.609, 24 p.186, 23 p.400-2]

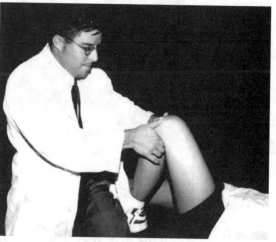

Anterior Drawer Test

B. Bounce Home Test

This test evaluates problems with full knee extension, usually due to meniscal tears or joint effusions. The patient is supine and the physician grasps the heel. The knee is flexed completely. Then, the knee is allowed to drop into extension. Normally, the knee should "bounce home" into full extension to a sharp end-point, without restriction. The test is positive if extension is incomplete or there is a "rubbery" feel to end-point extension. [23 p.413, 24 p.194]

C. Apley Compression and Distraction Tests

These tests evaluate the meniscus and ligamentous structures of the knee. The patient lies prone and the knee is flexed to 90°. The compression part of the test is performed with the physician pressing straight down on the heel, and internally and externally rotating the tibia in this position. Pain indicates a meniscal tear. Then, the physician pulls upward on the foot (the "distraction" part), and internally and externally rotates the tibia. Pain this time indicates ligamentous injury, usually the medial and/or lateral collateral ligaments. [24 p.193, 23 p.413]

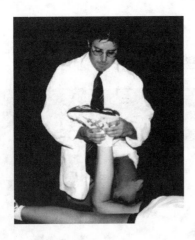

Apley's distraction test

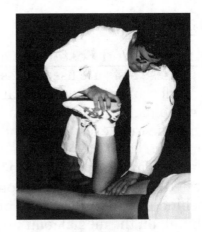

Apley's compression test

D. Lachman's Test

This test also assesses the stability of the ACL and is somewhat more accurate than the anterior drawer tests. The patient lies supine. The physician grasps the proximal tibia with one hand and the distal femur with the other hand. The knee is flexed to about 30°. The tibia is then pulled forward by the grasping hands. Both sides are compared, and the test is positive if the tibia excessively moves out from under the femur. [1 p.609, 23 p.397]

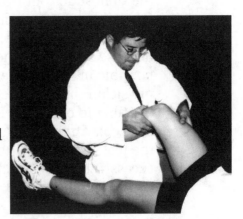

Lachman Test

E. McMurray Test

This test detects tears in the medial and lateral menisci of the knee. With the patient supine, the patient's knee is fully flexed. The physician's places on hand on the medial and lateral joint line of the knee and the other around the foot. The tibia is then externally rotated and a valgus stress is placed on the knee (see below left picture). Maintaining this position, the knee is then slowly extended. If a palpable or audible "click" is noticed, the test is positive for a tear of the meniscus. The test is repeated with internal rotation of the tibia and a varus stress on the knee(see below right picture). Again if a palpable or audible "click" is noticed, the test is positive for a tear of the meniscus. [1 p.630, 23 p.413, 24 p.191]

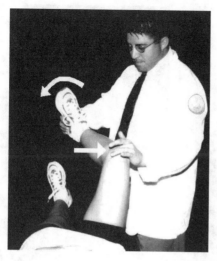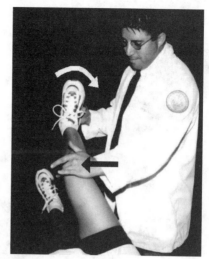

McMurray testing

F. Patellar Grind Test

This test assesses the posterior articular surfaces of the patella and the possibility of chondromalacia patellae, commonly seen with patello-femoral syndrome. The patient lies supine with knees fully extended and relaxed. The physician pushes the patella distally, then instructs the patient to contract the quadriceps muscles. Any roughness of the articular surfaces will grind, and be palpable and painful when the quadriceps contract and move the patella. The test is positive if the patient feels pain with contraction of the patella. [24 p.194, 23 p.418]

G. Valgus and Varus Stress Tests

These tests are used to assess the stability of the collateral ligaments. With the patient lying supine or sitting on the table, the knee is flexed just enough to unlock it from full extension. The physician stabilizes the ankle with one hand while the other pushes against the knee, first medially then laterally. Pushing the knee medially (with a **L**ateral force) is the va**L**gus stress test. If there is gaping on the opposite side, then the medial collateral ligament is torn. To test the lateral collateral ligament, the physician pushes the knee laterally (varus stress test). If there is any gaping of the lateral joint line, the test is positive.

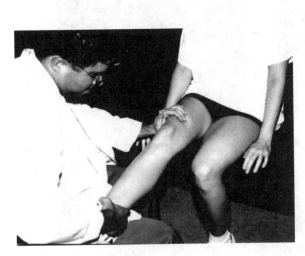

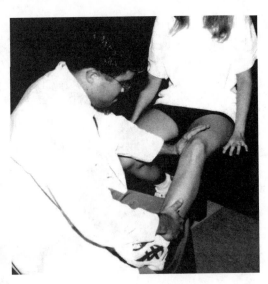

Valgus Stress Testing   *Varus Stress Testing*

VIII. Ankle

A. Anterior Draw Test of the Ankle

This test is used to assess the medial and lateral ligaments of the ankle, mainly the anterior talofibular ligament, but also the superficial and deep deltoid ligaments. The patient lies supine. The physician grasps the distal tibia/fibula with one hand, and pulls the foot forward with the other hand grasping the posterior aspect of the calcaneus. The foot should be held in 20° of dorsiflexion the entire time. If, after comparing both sides, excessive movement of the talus under the tibia/fibula occurs, then a bilateral injury has occurred to the mentioned ligaments. If there is deviation to one side, then only the ligaments to the opposite side of the foot are damaged. [23 p.480]

Chapter 18 Review Questions

1. A patient presents with left shoulder pain and an overuse injury is suspected. In order to evaluate shoulder range of motion you would perform the

   A. Adson test
   B. Apley compression test
   C. Apley distraction test
   D. Apley scratch test
   E. Roos test

2. A typist presents with chronic thumb pain on the radial side. History reveals the pain is worsened when holding objects. Examination reveals tenderness in the first dorsal compartment. Plain film radiography of the region is unremarkable. Which one of the following is most associated with the most likely diagnosis?

   A. it often results from repetitive and strenuous supination of the forearm
   B. it often requires procedural or surgical intervention
   C. it results from damage to the radial nerve
   D. it results from an inflammation of the abductor pollicis longus and/or extensor pollicis brevis tendons
   E. it results in a flexion contracture of the palmar fascia

3. A middle-aged female presents with nocturnal bilateral hand paresthesias and has a positive Phalen test. The most likely diagnosis is

   A. carpal tunnel syndrome
   B. de Quervain disease
   C. rotator cuff tear
   D. tennis elbow
   E. thoracic outlet syndrome

4. A patient with low back pain presents for evaluation. A hip drop test reveals that the left iliac crest drops 15 degrees with weightbearing on the right leg and the right iliac crest drops 25 degrees when weightbearing on the left leg. This test indicates that there is a

   A. congenital hip dislocation
   B. sidebending dysfunction of the lumbar spine
   C. sacral torsion
   D. sciatic nerve root compression
   E. inferior gluteal nerve neuropathy

5. A 15-year-old presents for a sports physical during which the Trendelenberg test is performed. This will assess the hip

    A. abductors
    B. adductors
    C. extensors
    D. external rotators
    E. flexors

6. A 45-year-old male presents to your office with left-sided low back pain. He states the pain is worsened by standing after a period of prolonged sitting. The pain reportedly radiates to his groin. On examination you notice that L1 is FR_LS_L with an associated tenderpoint medial to the left ASIS. You believe the problem lies within the left hip flexor. Which one of the following tests may aid in confirming your diagnosis?

    A. hip drop test
    B. Hoover test
    C. Ober test
    D. Thomas test
    E. Trendelenberg test

7. A 32-year-old female presents to the emergency department with acute knee pain after a basketball injury. Examination reveals effusion of the joint with a positive McMurray's test, and a positive Apley compression test. Apley distraction, anterior drawer, and valgus and varus tests are all negative. The most likely diagnosis is

    A. a medial collateral tear
    B. a medial meniscal tear
    C. a lateral collateral tear
    D. an anterior cruciate tear
    E. patellar chondromalacia

8. A 72-year-old female presents with low back pain after harvesting her garden. Observation reveals an elderly lady who is hunched forward. Physical exam reveals restriction of right thigh extension and a positive Thomas test on the right. Which of the following additional findings is most associated with this condition?

    A. anterior sacrum on the left
    B. pelvic side shift to the left
    C. positive spring test
    D. posterior sacrum on the right
    E. Trendelenberg test on the right

9. A 28-year-old male presents with acute low back pain. In the supine position you lift his right leg to 40 degrees with the knee extended when he experiences right-sided lumbar pain and right leg pain radiating below the knee. You then lift his left leg in the same manner and he again experiences right-sided lumbar pain and right buttock pain. The patient is most likely experiencing

    A. psoas pain
    B. sacroiliac pain
    C. lumbar degenerative disc disease
    D. sciatic nerve irritation
    E. lumbar facet syndrome

10. A patient has a positive standing flexion test on the right. This evaluates for

    A. iliosacral dysfunction
    B. lumbosacral dysfunction
    C. lumbosacral type II mechanics
    D. sacroiliac dysfunction
    E. sacropelvic unleveling

Questions 11-12 refer to the following:

A football player limps off the field reporting knee pain after an aggressive tackle. The athletic trainer assesses the knee and discovers excessive posterior movement of the tibia on the femur.

11. This is indicative injury to the

    A. ACL
    B. LCL
    C. MCL
    D. patellar tendon
    E. PCL

12. The patient then lies supine with the knee flexed at 90 degrees. The examiner compresses the knee into the table while internally and externally rotating the leg. Which one of the following statements is true concerning the Apley compression test? A pain response would indicate

    A. a meniscal injury
    B. both ligamentous and meniscal injury
    C. both posterior patellar surface and meniscal pathology
    D. ligamentous injury
    E. pathology on the posterior surface of the patella

Questions 13-14 refer to the following

For each numbered item (patient presentation) select one heading (diagnosis) most closely associated with it. Each lettered heading may be selected once, more than once, or not at all.

A. a rotator cuff tear
B. a flexion contracture of the iliopsoas
C. decreased muscle strength the gluteus medius
D. instability of the biceps tendon in the bicipital groove
E. thoracic outlet syndrome

13. A 45-year-old male laborer presents with shoulder pain and has a positive Adson test.

A. A
B. B
C. C
D. D
E. E

14. A 45-year-old female carpenter presents with upper extremity soreness and has a positive Yergason test.

A. A
B. B
C. C
D. D
E. E

Questions 15-16 refer to the following

For each numbered item (description) select one heading (special testing) most closely associated with it. Each lettered heading may be selected once, more than once, or not at all.

A. Adson test
B. Roos test
C. Speed test
D. Spurling test
E. Wallenberg test

15. Stenosis of the intervertebral foramen causing radiculopathy into the upper extremity can be most effectively assessed with

A. A
B. B
C. C
D. D
E. E

16. Which one of the following tests will be positive in vertebral artery insufficiency?

    A. A
    B. B
    C. C
    D. D
    E. E

Explanations

1. **Answer: D**

   Apley scratch test is used to evaluate the range of motion of the shoulder. To test abduction and external rotation, ask the patient to reach behind the head and touch the opposite shoulder. To evaluate internal rotation and adduction, ask the patient to reach in front of the head and touch the opposite shoulder. Next, to further evaluate internal rotation and adduction, instruct the patient to reach behind the back and touch the inferior angle of the opposite scapula. Observe the patient's movement for any asymmetry or any limitations of movement.

2. **Answer: D**

   This patient has de Quervain tendinopathy which affects both the abductor pollicis longus and extensor pollicis brevis muscles at the point where they pass through a fibrous tunnel (first dorsal compartment) from the forearm into the hand. Patients often have a positive Finkelstein test causing pain with wrist adduction when the patient makes a fist with the thumb tucked inside of the fingers. The condition is typically self-limited but may improve more quickly with a thumb spica splint and NSAIDs.

3. **Answer: A**

   The Phalen test evaluates for carpal tunnel syndrome during which the patient maximally flexes the wrist and holds this position for at least 60 seconds. This compresses the carpal tunnel and reproduces paresthesia symptoms. A common complaint in patients with carpal tunnel is parastheia that worsens with sleep.

4. **Answer: B**

   The question stem is describing a hip drop test. This test assesses the sidebending ability of the lumbar spine and thoracolumbar junction. With the patient standing, the physician locates the most superior and lateral aspect of the iliac crests. The patient is instructed to bend one knee without lifting the heel from the floor. Normally, the lumber spine should sidebend toward the side contralateral to the bending knee, producing a smooth convexity in the lumbar spine on the ipsilateral side. The ipsilateral iliac crest should drop more than 20-25°. A positive test is indicated by anything less than a smooth convexity in the lumbar spine, or a drop of the iliac crest of less than 20-25°, and alerts the physician to a somatic dysfunction of the lumbar or the thoracolumbar spine.[1 p.426]. Although sacral torsions and sciatic nerve root compression can be and often associated with structural asymmetries, the question is specifically asking about the hip drop test. Iliac crest asymmetry can also be seen with Trendelenberg testing. This test will be positive with hip abductor weakness (superior gluteal nerve). The inferior gluteal nerve innervates the gluteus maximus.

5. Answer: **A**

The Trendelenberg test assesses gluteus medius muscle strength. The gluteus medius is a hip abductor. The gluteus medius acts as a stabilizer during gait and prevents the unsupported iliac crest from dropping during the swing phase of gait. A weak gluteus medius is associated with fractures of the greater trochanter, slipped capital femoral epiphysis, lumbar somatic dysfunction, coxa vera, and nerve root lesions affecting muscle innervation.

6. Answer: **D**

This patient likely has a muscle strain or hypertonicity of the left iliopsoas muscle. The Thomas test assesses for flexion contracture of the hip which is most commonly associated with an iliopsoas spasm or contracture. If the iliopsoas muscle is shortened, the ipsilateral lower extremity will be unable to fully extend at the hip while in the supine position. The Hoover test is a maneuver aimed to separate organic from non-organic paresis of the leg. The patient is placed in a supine position. The physician places their hand under the patient's heel. The patient is then instructed to press the heels down onto the table. The examiner is expected to feel pressure on the non-paretic limb. The patient is then asked to raise their non-paretic limb against downward resistance applied by the physician. No pressure is expected to be felt under the paretic leg that is on the table. The Hoover sign is positive when pressure is felt the paretic leg when the non-paretic leg is raised and no pressure is felt in the non-paretic leg when the paretic leg is being raised.

7. Answer: **B**

The McMurray test detects tears in the posterior aspect of the menisci. The medial meniscus is tested with a valgus stress on the knee with external rotation while the lateral meniscus is tested with a varus stress on the knee with internal rotation.

8. Answer: **B**

Psoas syndrome is due to a psoas spasm that can cause a persistent strain across the lumbosacral junction and is associated with a constellation of signs and symptoms. The pelvic side shift test, like all somatic dysfunctions, is named positive to the side of freer motion. In a contracted psoas on the right, the pelvis will shift to the left resulting in a positive pelvic shift test to the left. Psoas syndrome is also associated with an L1 or L2 somatic dysfunction (not necessarily L5). Although some authors reported a sacral dysfunction on an oblique axis associated with psoas syndrome,[3] [p.747] sacral shear and posterior sacrum have not been reported. Other signs include flexed posture sidebent to the affected side, a positive Thomas test, enhanced lumbar lordosis, and tenderpoints of the ipsilateral iliacus and contralateral piriformis. [1 p.623]

9. Answer: **D**

The patient has a positive straight leg raise test, also known as Lasegue's sign/test. This is a nerve root test used to evaluate for sciatic nerve irritation. It is approximately 92% sensitive and 28% specific for disc herniation. The crossed straight leg raise test is positive when the pain is also reproduced in the affected leg with passive lifting of the unaffected side by the examiner; this is approximately 90% specific and 28% sensitive for disc herniation. The combination of the two for this patient is highly indicative of an acute disc herniation.

10. Answer: **A**

The standing flexion test assesses iliosacral motion. It evaluates the possibility of somatic dysfunction in the leg or pelvis, most commonly the innominate. [1 p.428] With the patient standing, the physician locates the patient's PSIS's and places his thumbs on the inferior notch. The patient is instructed to bend forward and the physician assesses the level of the PSIS's as this motion is completed. A positive test occurs when, at the termination of forward bending, the PSIS's are not level. Somatic dysfunction is present on the side of the superior PSIS.

11. Answer: **E**

The patient has a positive posterior drawer test consistent with injury to the posterior cruciate ligament (PCL). The PCL attaches anteriorly on the medial epicondyle of the femur and inserts onto the posterior intercondylar area of the tibia. If this is injured the femur may glide posteriorly on the tibia in an unstable fashion.

12. Answer: **A**

The Apley compression test assesses the menisci while the Apley distraction test assesses the ligaments (MCL and LCL).

13. Answer: **E**

The Adson test is performed while monitoring the patients distal radial pulse in an extended, externally rotated, and slightly abducted position. The patient is asked to take a deep breath and turn his/her head toward the ipsilateral arm. These motions further compress the neurovascular bundle and may cause a reduced or absent radial pulse consistent with thoracic outlet syndrome.

14. Answer: **D**

The Yergason test determines the stability of the biceps tendon in the bicipital groove. It is performed with the elbow flexed and having the patient resist external rotation while the physician also pulls downward on the patient's elbow. A positive test results when pain is elicited as the biceps tendon pops out of the bicipital groove.[24 p.32, 23 p.117]

15. Answer: **D**

The Spurling compression test can reproduce referred pain into the ipsilateral arm when compression is added to extension and sidebending of the cervical spine. This effectively narrows the intervertebral foramina and subsequently increases radicular complaints.

16. Answer: **E**

The Wallenberg test is performed in the supine position with the neck held in a flexed position for 10 seconds and then extended backward for 10 seconds. This is then repeated with the neck rotated to either side, then rotated while extended. A positive test is when the patient exhibits nystagmus or complains of dizziness or vision changes. Repeated or extreme cervical extension should be avoided for these patients due to the risk of vertebrobasilar sequelae with osteopathic manipulative techniques.

Common Techniques for Visceral and Systemic Dysfunctions

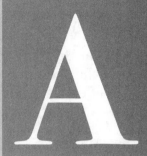

APPENDIX

Chapman's Reflexes [29 p.200, 20 p.64]

Objective - Decrease sympathetic tone, improve lymphatic return and increase myofascial motion associated with visceral dysfunction.

Indications - Visceral dysfunction

Sphenopalatine Ganglion Treatment [29 p.223, 20 p.232]

Objective - 1) Enhances parasympathetic activity which decreases goblet cells and thus encourages thin watery secretions. 2) Decongest the pterygoid fossa indirectly and improve nerve function of the sphenopalatine ganglion, thereby allowing normal function of the eustation tube. In addition, relaxation of the medial pterygoid muscle enables the tensor veli palatini muscle to relax to functionally open the eustachian tube.

Indications - Thick secretions associated with an upper respiratory tract infection (URI).

Rib Raising [29 p.195-98, 32 p.525]

Objective -
    Decrease sympathetic activity
    Improve negative intrathoracic pressure for maximum inhalation
    Improve lymphatic return

Indications -
    Hypersympathetic tone associated with visceral dysfunction
    Decreased respiration
    Fever
    Lymphatic congestion

Contraindications -
    Recent spinal surgery
    Rib fracture
    Spinal fracture

Paraspinal Inhibition

Procedure - Paraspinal pressure (similar to rib raising) at L1 and/or L2
Objective - Mainly used with rib raising to decrease sympathetic tone associated
    with an ileus
Indications - Ileus
Contraindications -
    Recent spinal surgery
    Rib fracture
    Spinal fracture

Celiac Ganglion Release [29 p.199-200]

Objective - Reduce sympathetic tone at T5 - T9
Indications - Upper GI dysfunction
Contraindications -
    Aortic aneurysm
    Nearby surgical wound

Superior Mesenteric Ganglion Release [29 p.199-200]

Objective - Reduce sympathetic tone at T10 - T11
Indications -
    GI dysfunction from jejunum to mid-transverse colon
    GU dysfunction
Contraindications -
    Aortic aneurysm
    Nearby surgical wound

Inferior Mesenteric Ganglion Release [29 p.199-200]

Objective - Reduce sympathetic tone at T12 - L2
Indications -
    Lower GI dysfunction
    GU dysfunction
    Pelvic dysfunction
Contraindications -
    Aortic aneurysm
    Nearby surgical wound

Sacral Rocking [1 p.774, 32 p.497]

Procedure - With the patient in the prone position, apply gentle pressure at the sacrum with rocking motion during inhalation and exhalation. The rocking motion augments flexion and extension phases associated with respiration or with the cranial rhythmic impulse (CRI).

Objective - Relaxes the muscles of the lumbosacral junction

Indications -
Tight lumbosacral paraspinals
Dysmenorrhea
Pelvic congestion syndrome
Sacroiliac dysfunction

Contraindications - Nearby infections or incisions

Thoracic Inlet Release [1 p.803, 32 p.518-19]

Objective - Improve lymphatic return in left and right lymphatic ducts.

Indications - Lymphatic congestion

Contraindications -
Upper rib fracture
Clavicle fracture
Lymphatic system malignancy

Redoming the Thoracoabdominal Diaphragm [1 p.803, 632p.526]

Objective - Increase thoracoabdominal diaphragm excursion improving respiration and improve lymph return.

Indications -
Decreased diaphragmatic excursion
Lymphatic congestion

Contraindications -
Local rib fracture
Nearby incision
Severe hiatal hernia or GERD
Lymphatic system malignancy

Pelvic Diaphragm Release

Objective - Improve pelvic diaphragm excursion and improve lymph return

Indications -
Decreased diaphragmatic excursion
Lymphatic congestion

Contraindications -
Local rib fracture
Nearby incision
Lymphatic system malignancy

Thoracic Pump [1 p.801, 32 p.523]

Objective - Augment thoracic range of motion and affect intrathoracic pressure
  gradients, improving lymphatic return
Indications -
  Lymphatic congestion
  Atelectasis
Contraindications -
  Osteoporosis (relative contraindication)
  Rib or spinal fracture
  Malignancy of lymphatic system

Pectoral Traction [32 p.524]

Objective - Augments thoracic range of motion via pectoralis minor stretch,
  improving lymphatic return. This technique facilitates the thoracic pump
Indications -
  Lymphatic congestion of the upper extremity
  Mild dyspnea or wheeze
  Reactive airway disease/asthma
Contraindications -
  Nearby surgical wound

Abdominal pump [3 p.1069]

Objective -
  Augments thoraco-abdominal pressure gradients improving lymphatic return
  Massages thoracic duct at cisterna chyli
Indications -
  Upper and lower GI dysfunctions
  CHF
  COPD, asthma, URI
  Hiatial hernia
  Decreased motion of L-spine and thoracic cage
Contraindications -
  Rib or spinal fracture
  Traumatic disruption of liver or spleen
  Nearby surgical incision
  A full stomach
  Lymphatic system malignancy

Liver and Spleen Pumps [1 p.801, 29 p.219-20]

Objective - Augments pressure gradient to improve lymphatic movement thus
  enhancing immune function and removing toxins

Indications -
    Right sided CHF
    Liver and splenic congestion
    Parenchymal disease of the liver and/or spleen
Contraindications -
    Spinal or rib fracture
    Acute hepatitis or friable liver
    Traumatic disruption of liver or spleen
    Lymphatic system malignancy

Pedal (Dalrymple) Pump [1 801, 35p. 218-19, 32 p.538]

Objective - Augments thoraco-abdominal pressure gradients improving lymphatic
    return.
Indications -
    Same as abdominal pump.
    Better suited in patients that cannot tolerate thoracic pump [29 p.229]
Contraindications -
    DVT
    Lower extremity fractures
    Recent abdominal surgery
    Acute ankle strain

Neurological Exam

I. Neurological evaluation:

A basic neurologic examination consists of muscle strength testing, sensation testing and deep tendon reflex testing. A detailed neurologic exam consisting of upper motor neuron signs is not in the scope of this text.

A. Muscle strength recording
Table B.1 shows the standard method for recording motor strength

Table B.1 [1 p.649]

Grade	Diagnosis	Definition
5	Normal	Full range of motion (FROM) against gravity and resistance
4	Good	FROM against gravity with some resistance
3	Fair	FROM against gravity with no resistance
2	Poor	FROM with gravity eliminated
1	Trace	Evidence of slight contractility
0	Zero	No evidence of contractility

B. Deep tendon reflex evaluation
Although differences may be subtle, table B.2 shows the standard way to record the amplitude of a reflex.[8 p.552]

Table B.2

Grade	Definition	Injury
4/4	Brisk with sustained clonus	Upper Motor Neuron
3/4	Brisk with unsustained clonus	Normal/UMN
2/4	Normal	Normal
1/4	Decreased but present	Normal/LMN
0/4	Absent	Lower Motor Neuron

II. Peripheral nerve distribution in the upper extremity

Table B.3 [23 p.50]

Nerve Root	Sensation	Motor	Reflex
C1	vertex of skull		none
C2	temple and occipital area		none
C3	supraclavicular fossa		none
C4	superior aspect of shoulder		none
C5	lateral aspect of elbow	elbow flexors	biceps reflex
C6	lateral forearm and thumb	wrist extensors	brachioradialis reflex
C7	middle finger	elbow extensors	triceps reflex
C8	little finger and middle forearm	deep finger and wrist flexors	none
T1	medial elbow and medial arm	finger abduction	none

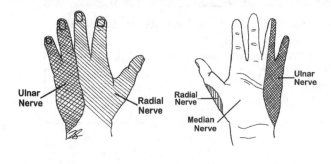

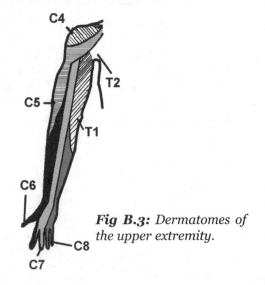

Fig B.3: *Dermatomes of the upper extremity.*

Figs B.1 and B.2: *Posterior (above left) and anterior (above right) view of the cutaneous distribution for the radial, ulnar, and median nerves.*

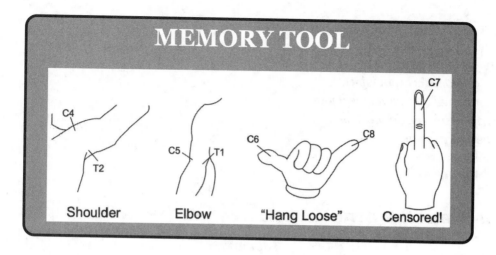

The above table and memory tool depicts dermatome locations as outlined in the International Standards for Neurological Classification of Spinal Cord Injury.[47]

III. Muscles of the shoulder

Table B.4

Muscle	Origin	Insertion	Innervation	Action
Deltoid	Lateral clavical, acromion, spine of scapula	Deltoid tuberosity of the humerus	Axillary nerve (**C5**, C6)	Abducts, adducts, flexes, extends shoulder
Supraspinatus	Supraspinous fossa of scapula	Gr. Tubercle of the humerus	Suprascapular nerve (C4,**C5**,C6)	Abducts arm
Infraspinatus	Infraspinous fossa of scapula	Gr. Tubercle of the humerus	Suprascapular nerve (C4,**C5**,C6)	Externally rotates arm
Subscapularis	Subscapula fossa	Lesser tubercle of the humerus	Upper and lower subscapular nerve (C5,**C6**,C7)	Internally rotates arm
Teres Major	Dorsal surface of inferior angle of scapula	Intertubercular groove of humerus	Lower sub scapular nerve (**C6**,C7)	Adducts and internally rotates arm
Teres Minor	Lateral border of scapula	Gr. Tubercle of the humerus	Axillary nerve (**C5**,C6)	Externally rotates arm
Lat. Dorsi	SP of T7 - T12, thoracolumbar fascia, iliac crest, ribs 9-12	Floor of bicipital groove of humerus	Thoracodorsal nerve (**C6,C7**,C8)	Adducts, extends shoulder Internally rotates arm

Table abbreviations
IO -= interosseous membrane
IP = Interphalangeal joint
CMC = carpometacarpal joint
PIP = proximal interphalangeal joint
DIP = distal interphalangeal joint
VB = vertebral body
SP = spinous process
IT = ischial tuberosity

IV. Muscles of the Arm

Table B.5

Muscle	Origin	Insertion	Innervation	Action
Coracobrachialis	Coracoid process of scapula	Middle third of medial surface of humerus	Musculocutaneous nerve (C5,**C6**,C7)	Flexes and adducts arm
Biceps brachii	*Long head*: Glenoid labrum, *Short head*: coracoid process	Radial tuberosity of radius	Musculocutaneous nerve (C5,**C6**)	Flexes elbow and supinates forearm
Brachialis	Lower anterior humerus	Coronoid proc. and ulnar tuberosity	Musculocutaneous nerve (C5,**C6**)	Flexes elbow
Triceps	Long Head: lateral edge of scapula Lateral head: humerus (superior to radial groove) Medial head: humerus (inferior to radial groove)	Olecranon process	Radial nerve (C6,**C7**,**C8**)	Extends elbow
Anconeus	Lateral epicondyle Proximal, median humerus	Olecranon process and ulna	Radial nerve (C7,C8,T1)	Extends elbow

VI. Muscles of the Anterior Forearm

Table B.6

Muscle	Origin	Insertion	Innervation	Action
Pronator teres	Medial epicondyle and coronoid process of ulna	Middle of lateral side of radius	Median nerve (C6,**C7**)	Pronates forearm
Flexor carpi radialis	Medial epicondyle	Base of 2nd and 3rd metacarpals	Median nerve (C6,**C7**)	Flexes and abducts hand
Palmaris longus	Medial epicondyle	Flexor retinaculum palmar aponeurosis	Median nerve (C7,C8)	Flexes hand
Flexor carpi ulnaris	Medial epicondyle and olecranon	5th metacarpal, pisiform, hamate	Ulnar nerve (C7,**C8**)	Flexes and adducts hand
Flexor digitorum superficialis	Medial epicondyle, coronoid process and radius	Middle phalanges (PIP's)	Median nerve (C7,**C8**,T1)	Flexes PIP's also flexes hand
Flexor digitorum profundus	Ulna and interosseous membrane	Distal phalanges (DIP's)	Median nerve (1 & 2 fingers)[**C8**,T1] Ulnar nerve (3 & 4 fingers)[C8,T1]	Flexes DIP's
Flexor pollicis longus	Radius, ulna and interosseous membrane	Distal phalanx of thumb	Median nerve (**C8**,T1)	Flexes thumb
Pronator quadratus	Anterior surface of distal ulna	Anterior surface of distal radius	Median nerve (**C8**,T1)	Pronates forearm

MEMORY TOOL

The **D**eep finger flexors (Flexor digitorum profundus) attach to the **DIPs.**

VII. Muscles of the Posterior Forearm

Table B.7

Muscle	Origin	Insertion	Innervation	Action
Brachioradialis	Supracondylar ridge of humerus	Base of radial styloid process	Radial nerve (C5,**C6**,C7)	Flexes forearm
Extensor carpi radialis longus	Supracondylar ridge of humerus	Base of 2nd metacarpal	Radial nerve (C6,C7)	Extends and abducts hand
Extensor carpi radialis brevis	Lateral epicondyle	Base of 3rd metacarpal	Radial nerve (**C7**,C8)	Extends and abducts hand
Extensor digitorum	Lateral epicondyle	Extensor expansion of PIP and DIP	Radial nerve (**C7**,C8)	Extends MCP's and wrist
Extensor digiti minimi	Lateral epicondyle	Extensor expansion of PIP and DIP of 5th digit	Radial nerve (**C7**,C8)	Extends 5th digit at PIP and DIP
Extensor carpi ulnaris	Lateral epicondyle and posterior ulna	Base of 5th metacarpal	Radial nerve (**C7**,C8)	Extends and adducts hand and wrist
Supinator	Lateral epicondyle, radial collateral and annular ligaments	Lateral proximal 3rd of radius	Radial nerve (C5,**C6**)	Supinates forearm
Abductor pollicis longus	Posterior radius, ulna and IO membrane	Base of 1st metacarpal	Radial nerve (C7,**C8**)	Abducts thumb and extends thumb at CMC
Extensor pollicis longus	Posterior ulna and IO membrane	Base of distal phalanyx of thumb	Radial nerve (C7,**C8**)	Extends IP and MCP of thumb
Extensor pollicis brevis	Posterior radius and IO membrane	Base of proximal phalanx of thumb	Radial nerve (C7,**C8**)	Extends CMC of thumb
Extensor indicis	Posterior ulna and IO membrane	Extensor expansion of PIP and DIP of 1st finger	Radial nerve (C7,**C8**)	Extends index finger

VIII. Muscles of the Hand

Table B.8

Muscle	Origin	Insertion	Innervation	Action
Abductor pollIcis brevis	Flexor retinaculum scaphoid and trapezium	Lateral side of proximal phalanx	Median nerve (**C8**,T1)	Abducts thumb
Flexor pollicis brevis	Flexor retinaculum trapezium	Lateral side of proximal phalanx	Median nerve (**C8**,T1)	Flexes thumb
Opponens pollicis	Flexor retinaculum and trapezium	Lateral side of 1st metacarpal	Median nerve (**C8**,T1)	Opposes thumb and other digits
Adductor pollicis	Capitate and 2nd, 3rd metacarpals	Medial side of proximal phalanx	Ulnar nerve (C8,**T1**)	Adducts thumb
Abductor digiti minimi	Pisiform	Medial proximal phalanx of 5th digit	Ulnar nerve (C8,**T1**)	Abduct little finger
Flexor digitorum mimimi brevis	Flexor retinaculum and hook of hamate	Medial proximal phalanx of 5th digit	Ulnar nerve (C8,**T1**)	Flexes PIP of little finger
Opponens digiti minimi	Flexor retinaculum and hook of hamate	Medial side of 5th metacarpal	Ulnar nerve (C8,**T1**)	Opposes little finger with thumb
Lumbricals	Flexor digitorum profundus tendon	Extensor expansions of fingers	Median nerve (1 & 2)(C8,**T1**) Ulnar nerve (3 & 4)(C8,**T1**)	Flexes MCP's and extends IP's
Dorsal interossi	Metacarpals	Extensor expansions and proximal phalanges	Ulnar nerve (C8,**T1**)	Abducts digits
Palmar interossi	Metacarpals	Extensor expansions and proximal phalanges	Ulnar nerve (C8,**T1**)	Adducts digits

IX. Peripheral nerve distribution in the lower extremity

Table B.9 [47]

Nerve Root	Sensation	Motor	Reflex
L1	anterior thigh just below inguinal ligament	hip flexors	none
L2	middle and anterior thigh	hip flexors & adductors	none
L3	anterior thigh just above knee	knee extensors	none
L4	**medial malleolus**	**ankle dorsiflexors**	**patella reflex**
L5	**dorsal aspect of foot and big toe**	**toe extensors**	none
S1	**lateral malleolus**	**ankle plantar flexors**	**achilles reflex**

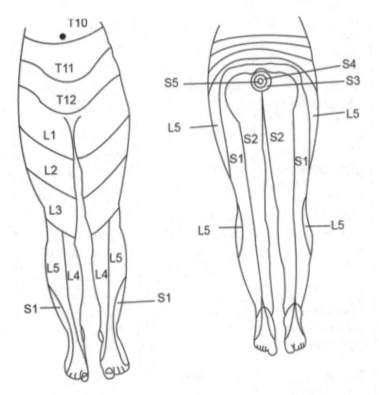

Fig B.4: *Dermatomes of the lower extremity*

X. Muscles of the Anterior Thigh

Table B.10

Muscle	Origin	Insertion	Innervation	Action
Iliopsoas	VB's of T12 - L5 and Iliac fossa	Lesser trochanter of femur	Femoral nerve (**L1, L2,** L3)	Flexes hip
Sartorius	ASIS	Upper medial side of tibia	Femoral nerve (L2 and L3)	Flexes abducts, and externally rotates thigh
Rectus femoris	AIIS and groove of acetabulum	Base of patella	Femoral nerve (L2, **L3, L4**)	Flexes hip and extends knee
Vastus medialis	Medial lip of femur	Base of patella	Femoral nerve (L2, **L3, L4**)	Extends knee
Vastus lateralis	Gr. trochanter and body of femur	Base of patella	Femoral nerve (L2, **L3, L4**)	Extends knee
Vastus intermedius	Body of femur	Base of patella	Femoral nerve (L2, **L3, L4**)	Extends knee

XI. Muscles of the Medial and Posterior Thigh

Table B.10

Muscle	Origin	Insertion	Innervation	Action
Adductor longus	Body of pubis	Middle 1/3 of linea aspera of femur	Obturator nerve (L2, **L3**, L4)	Adducts, flexes and internally rotates thigh
Adductor brevis	Body of inferior pubic ramus	Pectineal line, upper part of linea aspera	Obturator nerve (L2, **L3**, L4)	Adducts, flexes and internally rotates thigh
Adductor magnus	IT, inferior pubic ramus	Linea aspera, adductor tubercle, supracondylar line	Obturator and sciatic nerve (L2, **L3, L4**)	Adducts, flexes and extends thigh
Gracilis	Body and inferior pubic ramus	Superior part of medial tibia	Obturator nerve (**L2**, L3)	Adducts thigh, flexes leg
Semitendinosis	Ischial tuberosity (IT)	Superior part of medial tibia	Sciatic nerve, tibial portion (**L5, S1**, S2)	Extends thigh, flexes and internally rotates leg
Semimembranosis	Ischial tuberosity (IT)	Medial condyle of tibia	Sciatic nerve, tibial portion (**L5, S1**, S2)	Extends thigh, flexes and internally rotates leg
Biceps femoris	Long head: IT Short head: posterior femur	Head of fibula	Sciatic, LH = tibial, SH = peroneal (L5, **S1**, S2)	Extends thigh, flexes and externally rotates leg
Gluteus maximus	Ilium, sacrum, coccyx, sacrotuberus ligament	Gluteal tuberosity and iliotibial tract	Inferior gluteal nerve (**L5**, S1, S2)	Extends hip
Gluteus medius	Ilium	Greater trochanter	Superior gluteal nerve (**L5**, S1)	Abducts hip
Tensor fascia lata	Iliac crest and ASIS	Iliotibial tract	Superior gluteal nerve (L4, L5)	Flexes, abducts hip
Piriformis	Anterior sacrum and sacrotuberus ligament	Greater trochanter	Sacral nerve (**S1**, S2)	Externally rotates leg

XII. Muscles of the Anterior and Lateral Leg

Table B.12

Muscle	Origin	Insertion	Innervation	Action
Tibialis anterior	Lateral tibial condyle, IO membrane	1st cuneiform, 1st metatarsal	Deep peroneal nerve (**L4**, L5)	Dorsiflexes and inverts foot
Extensor hallucis longus	IO membrane, anterior fibula	Distal phalanx of big toe	Deep peroneal nerve (L5, S1)	Extends big toe, dorsiflexes foot
Extensor digitorum longus	Tibial condyle, IO membrane, fibula	Middle and distal phalanges	Deep peroneal nerve (L5, S1)	Extends digits 2-5, dorsiflexes foot
Peroneus longus	Lateral side and fibula head	base of 1st metatarsal, medial cuneiform	Superficial peroneal nerve (**L5**, **S1**, S2)	Everts and plantarflexes foot
Peroneus brevis	Lower lateral fibula	Base of 5th metatarsal	Superficial peroneal nerve (**L5**, **S1**, S2)	Everts and plantarflexes foot
Peroneus tertius	Distal 1/3 of fibula and IO membrane	Base of 5th metatarsal	Deep peroneal nerve (L5, S1)	Dorsiflexes and everts foot

XIII. Muscles of the Posterior Leg

Table B.13

Muscle	Origin	Insertion	Innervation	Action
Gastrocnemius	Lateral and medial femoral condyles	Posterior aspect of calcaneus	Tibial nerve (**S1**, S2)	Flexes knee, plantar-flexes foot
Soleus	Tibia and upper fibular head	Posterior aspect of calcaneus	Tibial nerve (**S1**, S2)	Plantar-flexes foot
Plantaris	Lower lateral supracondylar line	Posterior aspect of calcaneus	Tibial nerve (**L4**, **L5**, S1)	Weakly assists gastrocnemius
Popliteus	Lateral condyle of femur	Upper posterior side of tibia	Tibial nerve (**S2**, S3)	Unlocks knee and flexes knee
Flexor hallucis longus	Lower 2/3 of fibula, IO membrane	Distal phalanx of big toe	Tibial nerve (**S2**, S3)	Flexes great toe, plantar-flexes foot
Flexor digitorum longus	Middle posterior tibia	Base of distal phalanges	Tibial nerve (L4, L5)	Flexes toes 2-5, plantar-flexes foot
Tibialis posterior	IO membrane, proximal tibia and fibula	Navicular, cuneiforms, cuboid, metatarsals 2-4 Tibial nerve (S1, S2)		Plantar-flexes and inverts foot.

XIV. Muscles of the Foot

Table B.14

Muscle	Origin	Insertion	Innervation	Action
Extensor digitorum brevis	Dorsal surface of calcaneus	Tendons of extensor digitorum longus	Deep peroneal nerve (L5,S1)	Extends toes
Extensor hallucis brevis	Dorsal surface of calcaneus	Proximal phalanyx of big toe	Deep peroneal nerve (L5,S1)	Extends big toe
Abductor hallucis	Medial tubercle of calcaneus	Proximal phalanyx of big toe	Medial plantar nerve (S2,**S3**)	Abducts and flexes big toe
Flexor digitorum brevis	Medial tubercle of calcaneus	Middle phalanyx of toes 2-5	Medial plantar nerve (S2,**S3**)	Flexes middle phalanx of toes 2-5
Abductor digiti minimi	Medial and lateral tubercles of calcaneus	5th proximal phalanyx	Lateral planter nerve (S2,**S3**)	Abducts little toe
Quadratus plantae	Medial and lateral surface of calcaneus	Tendon of flexor digitorum longus	Lateral planter nerve (S2,**S3**)	Assists flexor digitorum in flexing toes
Lumbricals	Tendons of flexor digitorum longus	Proximal phalanges of 2-5 and extensor expansion	Medial and lateral planter nerves (S2,**S3**)	Flexes proximal phalanges & extend distal phalanges of toes 2-5
Flexor hallucis brevis	Cuboid and lateral cuneiform	Proximal phalanx of big toe	Medial plantar nerve (S1,**S2**)	Flexes big toe
Adductor hallucis	Distal and proximal metatarsals	Proximal phalanx of big toe	Lateral plantar nerve (S2,**S3**)	Adducts big toe
Flexor digiti minimi brevis	Base of 5th metatarsal	Proximal phalanx of little toe	Lateral plantar nerve (S2,**S3**)	Flexes little toe
Plantar interossei	Medial sides of metatarsals 3-5	Medial base of proximal phalanges of 3-5	Lateral plantar nerve (S2,**S3**)	Adducts toes and flexes MTP's
Dorsal interossei	Adjacent sides of metatarsals	Base of proximal phalanx 2-4	Lateral plantar nerve (S2,**S3**)	Abducts toes and flexes MTP's

REFERENCES

1. American Osteopathic Association: Foundations for Osteopathic Medicine. Third Edition. Philadelpia, LippencottWilliams and Wilkins, 2011.

2. DiGiovanna, E., Schiowitz, S.: An Osteopathic Approach to Diagnosis and Treatment. Third Edition Philadelphia, Lippencott Williams and Wilkins, 2005

3. American Osteopathic Association: Foundations for Osteopathic Medicine. 2nd Edition. Baltimore, Lippencott, Williams and Wilkins, 2002

4. Thorpe, RG: Manipulative procedures in Lumbosacral Problems, Osteopathic Annals, August 1974

5. Moore, K.L.: Clinically Oriented Anatomy. Third Edition. Baltimore, Williams and Wilkins, 1992.

6. Bland, J.H.: Disorders of the Cervical Spine: Diagnosis and Medical Management. Second Edition. Philadelphia, W.B. Saunders, 1994

7. Kuchera, W.A., Kuchera, M.L.: Osteopathic Principles in Practice. Second Edition (revised), second printing, Colum- bus, Greyden Press, 1993.

8. American Osteopathic Association: Foundations for Osteopathic Medicine. Baltimore, Williams and Wilkins, 1997.

9. Moore, K.L.: Clinically Oriented Anatomy. Third Edition. Baltimore, Williams and Wilkins, 1992

10. Kimberly, P.E., Funk, S.L.: Outline of Osteopathic Manipulative Procedures: The Kimberly Manual. Millennium Edi- tion. Walsworth Publishing Co, 2000

11. Boden, SD et.al.: Orientation of lumbar facet joints: Association with Degenerative Disc Disease. Journal of Bone and Joint Surgery. March 1996: 78-A(3) p.403 - 411

12. Brashear, Jr, H.R., Raney, Sr, R.B.: Handbook of Orthopaedic Surgery. Tenth Edition. St. Louis, C.V. Mosby Co., 1986

13. Goldberg, S: Clinical Anatomy Made Ridiculously Simple. MedMastor. Inc., 1984

14. DiGiovanna, E., Schiowitz, S.: An Osteopathic Approach to Diagnosis and Treatment. Philadelphia, J.B. Lippencott Co., 1991.

15. Borenstein, D.G., Wiesel, S.W., Boden, S.D.: Low Back Pain. Second Edition. Philadelphia, W.B. Saunders Co., 1995

16. Deyo, R.A., Diehl, A.K., Rosenthal M.: How many days of bed rest for acute low back pain? A randomized clinical trial. New England Journal of Medicine. Oct 1986: 23;315(17):1064-70

17. Snider, R.K.: The Essentials of Musculoskeletal Care. American Academy of Orthopedic Surgeons, 1997

18. Buckwalter, J.A., Weinstein, S.L.: Turek's Orthopaedics: Principles and their Applications. Fifth Edition. Philadelphia, J.B. Lippincott Co.

19. Anderson, D.M.: Dorland's Illustrated Medical Dictionary. 28th Edition. Philadelphia, WB Saunders, 1994

20. Nelson, K.E, Gloneck, T.: Somatic Dysfunction in Osteopathic Family Medicine. Second Edition. Wolters Kluwer, 2015

21. DiGiovanna, E., Schiowitz, S.: An Osteopathic Approach to Diagnosis and Treatment. Second Edition. Philadelphia, J.B. Lippencott Co., 1997.

22. Berkow, R.: Merck Manual. Sixteenth Edition. Rahway, Merck Research Laboratories, 1992

23. Magee, D.J.: Orthopedic Physical Assessment. Second Edition. Philadelphia, W.B. Saunders Co., 1992

24. Hoppenfeld, S: Physical Examination of the Spine and Extremities. Norwalk, Appleton-Century-Crofts, 1976

25. Rubin, A., Stallis, R.: Evaluation and Diagnosis of Ankle Injuries. American Family Physician. 1996;54(5):1609-1618

26. www.ncbi.nlm.nih.gov/pubmed/1550645 www.ncbi.nlm.nih.gob/pubmed/1962712

27. Magoun, H.I.: Osteopathy in the Cranial Field. Kirksville, The Journal Printing Co., 1976

28. Greenman, P.E.: Principles of Manual Medicine. Second Edition. Baltimore, Williams and Wilkins, 1996

29. Kuchera, W.A., Kuchera, M.L.: Osteopathic Considerations in Systemic Dysfunction. Second Edtion (revised). Columbus, Greyden Press, 1994

30. Frymann, V.M.: The Collected Papers of Voila M. Frymann, DO: Legacy of Osteopathy to Children. Indianapolis, American Academy of Osteopathy, 1998

31. Dambro, M.R.: Griffith's Five-Minute Clinical Consult 2000. Eighth edition. Lippincott, Williams and Wilkins 2000

32. Nicholas, A.S: Atlas of Osteopathic Techniques. Third Edition, Wolters Kluwer 2016

33. Jones, L.H.: Jones Strain-Counterstrain. Jones Strain-Counterstrain inc., Boise, 1995

34. Patterson, M.M.: A model mechanism for spinal segmental facilitation. JAOA. 1976;76:62/121-72/131.

35. Fix, J.D.: Neuroanatomy. Second Edition. Baltimore, Williams and Wilkins, 1995

36. Berne, R., Levy, M: Physiology. Third edition. St. Louis, Mosby, 1993.

37. Guyton, A.: Textbook of Medical Physiology. Eighth Edition. Philadelphia, W.B. Saunders 1991.

38. Owens, C.: An Endocrine Interpretation of Chapman's Reflexes, 1937. Reprinted by the Academy of Applied Os- teopathy, May 1963.

39. Travell, J.G., Simons, D.G.: Myofascial Pain and Dysfunction. Vol I. Baltimore, Williams and Wilkins, 1983.

40. Travell, J.G., Simons, D.G.: Myofascial Pain and Dysfunction. Vol II. Baltimore, Williams and Wilkins, 1983

41. Simons, D.G.: Muscle Pain Syndromes. Journal of Manual Medicine. 1991:6:3-23

42. Chaitow, L.: Soft Tissue Manipulation. Ellington, Great Britian, Thorston Publishing, 1987.

43. Gray's Anatomy. 38th Edition. New York Edinburgh London Tokyo Madrid and Melbourne, Churchill Livingston, 1995.

44. Yates, H.A., Glover, J: Counterstrain: A Handbook of Osteopathic Technique. Tulsa, Y-Knot Publishers, 1995.

45. Mitchell, F.L., Moran P.S., Pruzzo N.A..: An Evaluation and Treatment Manual of Osteopathic Muscle Energy Proce- dures. First Edition. Mitchell, Moran & Pruzzo Associates, 1979

46. Neer CS 2nd. Impingement lesions. Clin Orthop Relat Res. 1983 Mar;(173):70–7

47. Marino, R.J.: International Standards for Neurological Classification of Spinal Cord Injury. 6th edition. American Spinal Injury Association, 2002

A

G

Goblet cells 181, 300
Golfers elbow (see Medial epicondylitis)
Golgi tendon organs 237, 255
Gracilis muscle 314

Hamate bone 115
Hamstrings 131, 135, 281
    Tightness of 56, 84
    (see also individual muscles)
Hand
    Anatomy 114
    Blood supply 108
    Deformities 120
    Joints 115
    Muscles 115
    Sensation 306
Head and neck
    Lymphatic drainage 211
    Sympathetic innervation 170
Headache 163
Hearing loss 160
Heart
    Autonomic effects on 177
    Failure (see Congestive heart failure)
    Lymphatic drainage 211
    Parasympathetic innervation 178
    Sympathetic innervation 179
    Trigger point and 195
Heat 52
Heel lift (see Short leg syndrome)
Heel spur 141
Hemophilia 257
Hepatitis 304
Hernia
    Hiatal 303
Herniated disc
    (see Nucleus pulposus, herniated)
High velocity, low amplitude (HVLA) 255-564
    Cervical spine 257-259
    Contraindications 11, 52, 54, 256, 277
    General procedure 256
    Indications 256
    Lumbar spine 52, 54, 262-264
    Neurophysiologic mechanism 255
    Rib dysfunction 261-262
    Thoracic spine 259-261
Hip
    Anatomy 131
    Deformity 135
    Examination 285, 286
    Fracture 71
    Joints 132
    Ligaments 132
    Motion of 132
    Muscles of 131

    Nerves 135
    In scoliosis 70
    Screening tests of 183, 285, 286
    Somatic dysfunction 134
Hip drop test 281
Hospitalized patients and OMT 11
Humerus 103, 113, 115
    Fracture 114
HVLA (see High velocity, low amplitude)
Hyoid 216
Hyperabduction test (see Hyperextension test)
Hyperextension test 112, 278
Hypertension
    Lymphatic effects 214
Hypoalbuminemia
    Lymphatic effects 214
Hypoglossal canal 160

Ice 52
Idiopathic scoliosis 69
Ileus
    Prevention treatment 182, 301
Iliac crest 49, 68, 281
Iliacus muscle 135, 230
Iliopsoas muscle 49, 131, 132
    Somatic dysfunction (see Psoas syndrome)
    (see also Psoas muscle and Iliacus muscle)
Iliosacral joint
    Assessing motion 282
Iliotibial tract
    Chapman's point 194
    Ober's test 285
Ilium 79
Immune function 303
Incontinence 58
Indirect techniques
    Vs. Direct 9, 10
    When to use 11
    (see also specific treatment types or specific areas of the spine)
Infection
    As a cause of back pain 51
    As a cause of scoliosis 69
    In lymphatic treatment 217
Inferior gluteal nerve 314
Inferior lateral angles (ILA's) (see Sacrum, landmarks)
Inflare, innominate (see Innominate, *somatic dysfunction*)

Lift therapy (see short leg syndrome)
Ligaments
  Alar 21
  Ankle 140-141
  Anterior cruciate 132, 287, 288
  Anterior talofibular 140, 214, 290
  Calcanofibular 140
  Calcaneonavicular 140
  Capitus femoris 132
  Cervical 21
  Deltoid 141
  Fibular collateral (lateral collateral) 133, 289
  Iliofemoral 132
  Iliolumbar 80
     Stress and 70, 80
  Injury 138
  Ischialfemoral 132
  Lateral collateral (knee) 133, 289
  Ligamentum flavum 54
  Medial collateral (knee) 133, 138, 289
  Of Treitz 181
  Pelvic
     Accessory 80
     True 80
  Plantar 141
  Posterior cruciate 133, 287
  Posterior longitudinal 48, 53, 54
  Posterior talofibular 140
  Pubofemoral 132
  Sacroiliac 70, 80
  Sacrospinous 80
  Sacrotuberous 80
     Tension of in dysfunction 80
  Sprain
     Degrees of 138
  Spring (see Calcaneonavicular)
  Talofibular
     Anterior 140
     Posterior 140
  Tibial collateral (medial collateral) 133, 138, 289
  Transverse 21, 256

Liver
  Autonomic effects on 177
  Lymphatic drainage 212
  Parasympathetic innervation 178
  Spleen pump 216, 303
  Sympathetic innervation 179
Long thoracic nerve 109, 114
Lordosis, lumbar 56, 287
Loss of motion
  In somatic dysfunction 2
Louis, angle of 34
Low velocity, moderate amplitude
  techniques (see Articulatory techniques)
Lower extremity
  Anatomy 131, 139
  Joints 132, 139
  Ligaments 131
  Muscles 131
  Innervation 132
  Somatic dysfunction 132, 136, 137, 140
  Sympathetic innervation 179
  (See also Ankle; Hip; Knee; etc)
Lumbar lordosis (see lordosis)

Lumbar spine 48
  Anatomy 48
  Anatomical variations 49
  Counterstrain 230
  Discs 48
     Herniated (see Nucleus pulposus, herniated)
  Effect on psoas 49,52
  Effect on sacrum (see Lumbar spine, rules of L5
  Examination 6, 282
  Facet joints 7, 49, 54
  Findings in scoliosis 70
  Herniated discs (see Nucleus pulposus, herniated)
  HVLA of 262-264
  Intervertebral foramen 48, 54
  Lamina 50
  Ligaments of 48
  Manipulation11 (see also specific treatment types)
  Motion of 50
  Muscle energy 244
  Nerves 48
  Pain (see Pain, lumbar)
  Rules of L5 51, 88
  Screening test (see also Hip drop test)
  Somatic dysfunction 50
  Spondylolisthesis (see Spondylolisthesis)
  Spondylolysis (see Spondylolysis)
  Stenosis 54
  Transverse processes 48
Lumbarization 50
Lumbosacral
  Angle (see Ferguson's angle)
  Decompensation 80
  Joint 51
  Junction 205
  Spring test 89,284
Lumbricals
  Foot 317
  Hand 311
Lunate bone 115
Lungs
  Autonomic effects on 177
  Chapman's points 193
  Lymphatic drainage 211
  Parasympathetic innervation 178
  Sympathetic innervation 179
Luschka, Joints of 21, 25
  In nerve root compression 21, 25
Lymph system 211-218
  Anatomy 211
  Anatomicophysiologic relationships 212
  Fluid
     Factors influencing movement 213
  Innervation 213
Lymphatic drainage
  Right (minor) duct 108,211,216
  Left (main) duct 108, 211, 216
  Thoracic duct 211,212,216
  (see also Thoracic duct)
Lymphatic dysfunction
  Congestion 300, 302, 303

Yergason's test 279

Zink D.O., J. Gordon 205
Zygapophyseal joints
  Cervical spine 21
        In nerve root compression 21, 25
  Orientation 7, 8, 256
  Tropism (see tropism)